CLEAVED

A story of loss, legs and finding family

JANE CAFARELLA

Published by Jane Cafarella
Melbourne, Australia
janecafarella.com.au

First published 2024
Copyright © Jane Cafarella, 2024

The moral rights of the author have been asserted.

All rights reserved. This book is copyright. Apart from any fair dealing for the purpose of private study, research, ciriticism or review as permitted under the *Copyright Act*, no part may be reproduced by any process without written permission. Inquiries should be made to the publisher.

Some names have been changed to protect the identities and privacy of people still living.

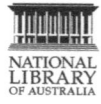 A catalogue record for this book is available from the National Library of Australia

ISBN: 978 1 7635081 0 1 (pbk)

Cover design: Bradley Dawson (Smith and Brown Design) and Jane Cafarella
Cover image: The author and her sister Juliana aged 7 and 8 respectively, with their mother – from the author's private collection
Author image: Leonie Van Eyk Photography
Typesetting: Helen Christie (Blue Wren Books)

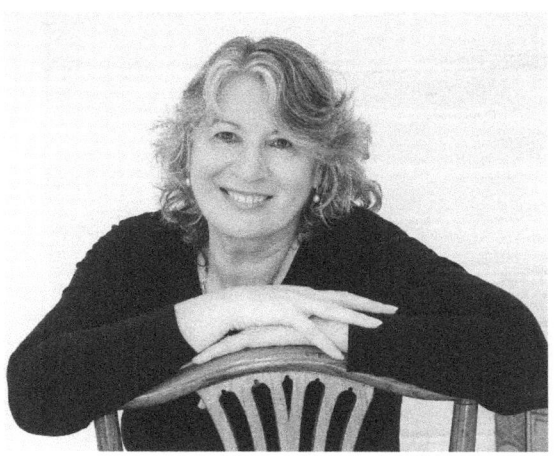

Jane Cafarella is an Australian playwright and former journalist and cartoonist whose work has been widely published in Australia and overseas and whose plays have been performed nationally and internationally. Her cartoon archive is held at the State Library of Victoria.

During her 10 years at Melbourne's *Age* newspaper, Jane wrote and edited the popular *Accent* section, which focused on women's issues, and for many years wrote the beloved columns *A New Life Journal* and *Family Postcard*.

What she didn't write about was growing up with what she later discovered was Milroy's disease, a rare form of the incurable and progressive swelling disease lymphoedema – and how she came to be estranged from her family of origin for most of her adult life.

When she did, it changed her life.

Here's what readers like you are saying about CLEAVED:

"… I can't put it down. It's warm, honest, brilliant."
—Jan Harkin, Victoria

"I can't put into words how much I enjoyed your book!"
—Sheralyn Iljcesen, South Australia

"I just finished it. I'm in bits. Such a beautiful story."
—Susie Penrice Tyrie, Singapore

"Honestly you've touched every emotion
and feeling in my heart."
—Magdalini Lazarro, Victoria

"I practically inhaled your book – I found it such
a fascinating story, beautifully written."
—Jane Haley, Tasmania

For my children and grandchildren

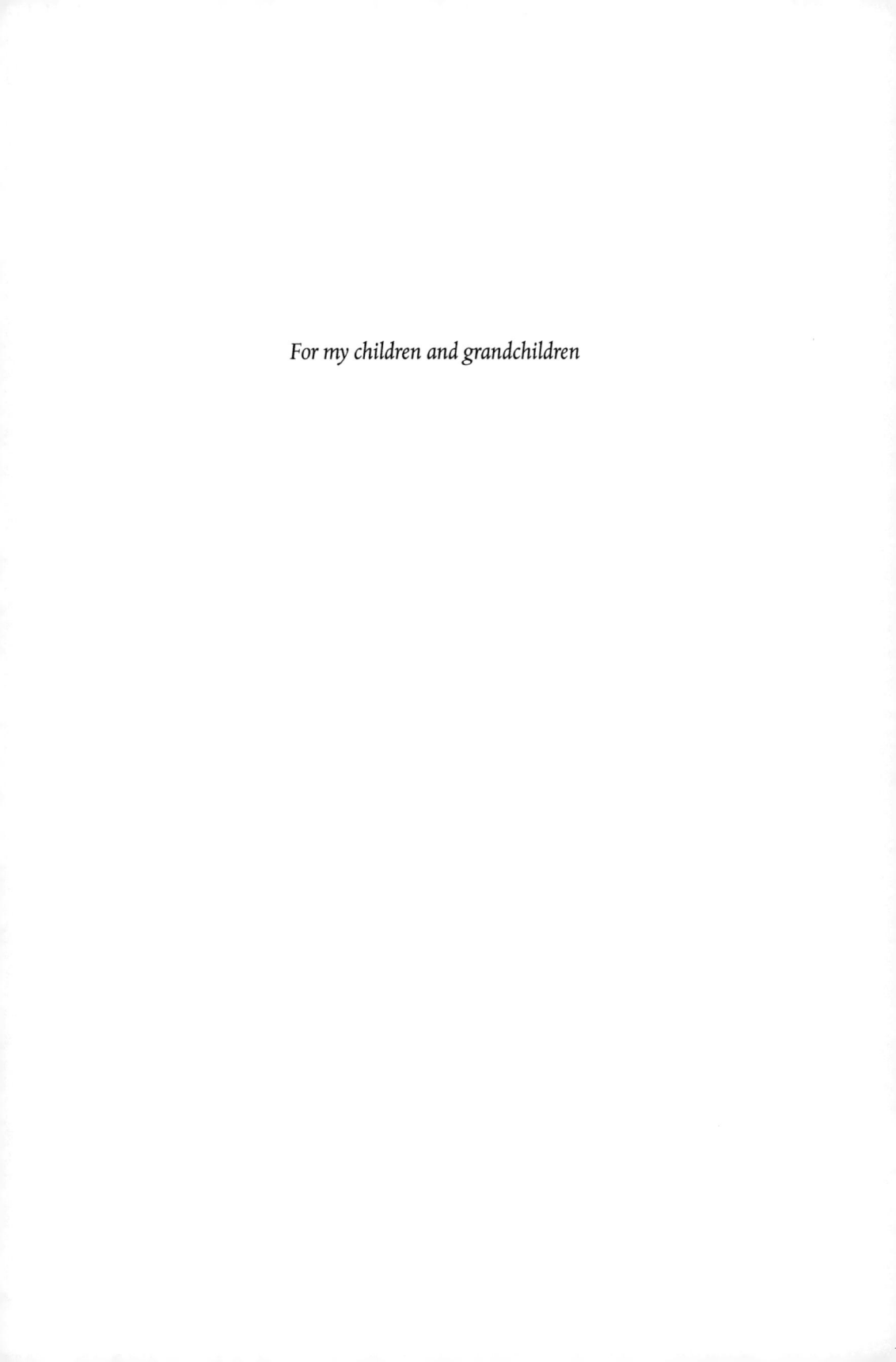

The World Health Organisation estimates that up to 250 million people worldwide live with the incurable, disfiguring, progressive, and little-known disease called lymphoedema. In Jane Cafarella's new memoir, CLEAVED, the veil of secrecy surrounding lymphoedema is stripped away as we meet a young girl in Australia living with an undiagnosed deformity. Ms Cafarella weaves a stirring and universal coming-of-age story where the audience gets a rare glimpse of the impact of living with a disability while traversing the many roads on life's journey.

—William Repicci, CEO of the Lymphatic Education and Research Network (NYC)

Cleave (intransitive verb): to adhere firmly, closely, loyally and unwaveringly,

Cleave (transitive verb): to split forcefully, to separate into distinct parts, and especially into groups having divergent views.

Contronym: a word that has two meanings that contradict one another.

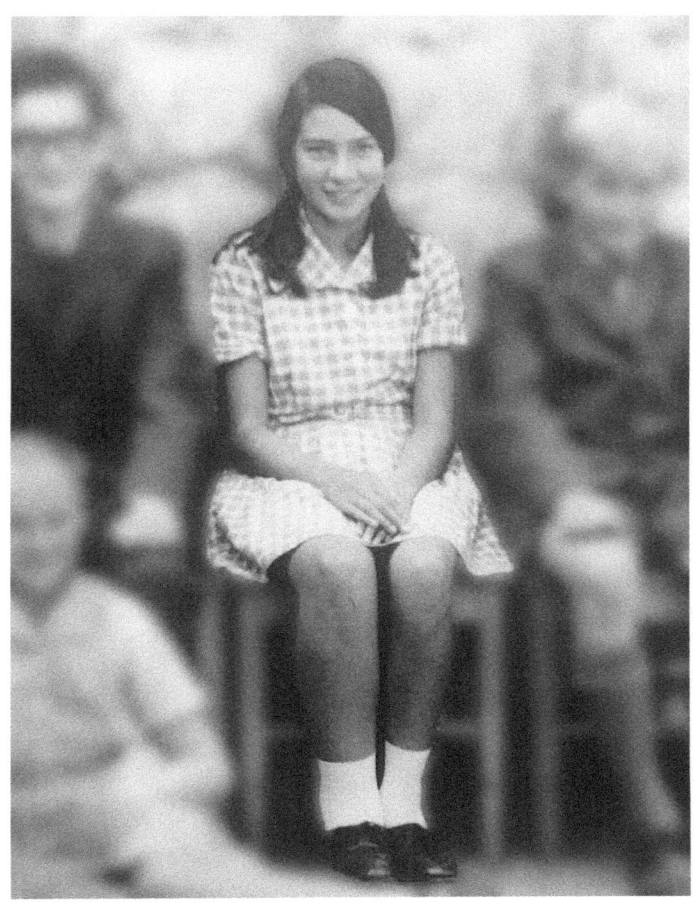

Me at age 13 in high school. This was the last photo I allowed that showed my leg. I soon learned to sit at the back. Later, as it worsened, I wore long dresses or flares to hide it.

PART ONE

Cleaving

1

Parkdale, 1974

The jagged nail on the ring finger of my left hand is proof that my sister Julie hates me, or so my mother tells me.

"You were just a baby," she says, puffing on her cigarette. "We were living in Croydon. I heard you crying and found you sitting up in the pram with blood all over your hand. You'd been sitting with your fingers on the edge of the pram when Julie brought the hood down on them.

"Your father was at work. Croydon was just the sticks then. I had no car and no phone. I gathered you up and started running, running, running, with Julie clinging to my skirts, across the paddocks to the neighbour's house to call the doctor," she says, panting in recollection.

Instinctively, I curl my fingers into my palm and examine my nail, painted pearly pink, and the scar, barely detectable now, where the dangling finger was sewn back.

"She's perverse," my mother says, reaching for the sherry bottle and pouring a preparatory glass – Three Roses, her favourite.

I am 17. I sit opposite on a kitchen chair across the wobbly card table in our tiny flat with its big square window, masked by a squinting venetian blind drawn against the cold of a winter evening. She is 47. Her dark wispy hair is drawn back from her long pale face in a bun.

Her skin is still smooth but her full mouth is empty of smiles. She wears no make-up, except for red lipstick, transferred to the filter of the cigarette she holds. There's no one to impress except me, and I'm already on her side.

The story of the pram and the blood is the sequel to the main story, which I know is next – of how my sister and I were separated at birth, although we grew up in the same house.

My mother sips and sighs and begins to speak in the low seductive voice of a seasoned storyteller, the voice of a singer who has been trained and whose words carry across rooms and decades.

I don't listen. I don't have to. Like all her stories, I know this one by heart.

**

1956

It was a cold winter day in July. My mother lay in the hospital bed next to my sister's crib. It had been a difficult birth. Her first pregnancy had been ectopic – the foetus aborting after implanting in the fallopian tube. By the time this second pregnancy reached full term her Rh-negative Rhesus "monkey blood", as she called it, had developed a battalion of antibodies, poisoning my sister's Rh-positive blood and turning her into a "blue baby". A blood transfusion saved her life. Shocked and exhausted, my mother lay waiting to be comforted and consoled. But the new father wasn't interested in the new mother.

"He walked straight past me to the crib and picked her up, and I thought, she's his," she tells me, describing again how she and my father sealed my sister's fate.

The only claim my mother makes to the child is to name her Juliana Sophia, after her maternal great grandmother, who is of Danish heritage. The beautiful musical name, the perfect accompaniment to Cafarella – my father's Italian surname – is recorded on the baptism certificate, but at home she is just Julie, the child of the father who claims her and renames her.

Fourteen months later, I am born – six weeks early, as the battalion of antibodies in my mother's blood has become an army.

"You were two pounds and the colour of that table," she tells me every birthday, pointing to our mahogany dining table. I am transfused twice. My lungs are as tiny and fragile as butterfly wings. There are no guarantees, the doctor says. A priest is summoned, along with a miracle. When it's granted, I am the child my mother claims.

"I cleaved you to me. I grabbed you up, because you were a very ill baby," she tells me as the years roll by, her jade eyes wide. "I was around you all the time, weeping and crying. Around you all the time, stuck to you like glue."

And the story of our cleaving feels both inevitable and uncomfortable, a fairy tale curse – and a gift.

She names me Jane Louise after her father Lewis and his mother Jane. Yorkshire pudding followed by Spaghetti Bolognese. Unmusical. My father doesn't comment.

Not long after my severed finger heals, I am crawling around the floor of the doctor's office where Mum has taken me for my check-up.

"Notice anything about her?" the doctor says.

"Yes," Mum says. "She's beautiful."

"What else?" asks the doctor.

"Nothing else."

"Look at her legs."

"What about them?"

"One is bigger."

My right leg, from calf to foot, is indeed slightly bigger than the left. Mum also suffers from puffy feet. But this is different. It never goes down. There's no name and no treatment, the doctor says. I am just born that way, so it's ignored. I can walk, and run, although over the years, it gets bigger and my foot prickles and aches and swells further in the heat, spilling over the edges of my shoe like a cake baked in a tin that's too small. My mother cleaves me further, and the chasm between my sister and me grows a little wider.

The black-and-white photo of Julie aged three standing in Dad's work boots is proof of our allegiances. She wears baggy overalls and an unflattering pudding-bowl haircut, accentuating her broad face and wide-spaced amber-green eyes, a darker shade of Mum's. Her hair is brown and her skin is fair like Mum's, while I have Dad's olive skin and the dark eyes of the grandfather I am named after. My hair is dark and wispy like Mum's, except mine forms floppy curls. Mum licks her finger and twists the curls around it to make them stick.

***

While Dad is focused on getting rich in the milk bar business, Mum makes us her projects. She dubs me Pebble-head, for my oval face, and Julie Pumpkin-top, for her round face, and pins tiny cotton bags containing camphor squares to our singlets, to ward off colds. She dresses us in the little cotton pinafores that her mother, Nanny, makes, with matching ribbons in our hair.

"You had little brown boots that I polished till they shone," she tells me, except where Julie has one pair I have two for my mismatched feet.

She saves up for a double pusher with a fringe of pompoms around the hood, and pushes us triumphantly down the street, the little blue babies who are now pink and bonny (or in my case, brown): testament to her struggle and sacrifice. "Are they twins?" strangers gush, although anyone can see we're not. We are too different.

I am three and Julie is four when Perry, Dad's partner in the milk bar business, is jailed for fraud, although I am never told Perry's full name or what sort of fraud he committed. Unable to pay his debts, Dad is declared bankrupt, though Mum says he probably could have managed that all by himself.

"He used to lock all the bills in the desk and refuse to open them," she says.

The stench of shame follows us a year later when we move from "the sticks" in Croydon to a three-bedroom weatherboard house in

Remo Street, in the bayside suburb of Mentone. Our house in Remo Street is a short walk from Nanny and Pa's house in Florence Street, and Dad's sister Mary in Balcombe Road, where the conversations are peppered with Sicilian dialect, which everybody understands except Mum, Julie and me. Like Mentone, where all the main streets are named after Italian towns and cities, we are fake Italians in fake Italy.

"Can we swing on your muscles?" Julie says, skipping towards Dad as he walks towards us along Mentone Parade one summer evening on the way home from work, his brown shoulders bare under the loose bib of his paint-spattered blue overalls. He puts his hands behind his head, flexing his muscles until they form hard hills. Julie hangs on, but I hang back. Though she's a year older, she is lighter, as my leg weighs heavy. Encouraged by Mum, I join her and the smell of putty, paint, motor oil, cigarettes and PK chewing gum greets me as I lift my legs and swing briefly, before Dad drops his arms.

Today he is a spray painter, with rags streaked with pink putty poking from his pockets. Sometimes he's a welder, and his bright blue eyes are red from the bits of metal that fly into them. Sometimes, he works nightshift in a factory as a fitter and turner, although I don't know what he fits or turns. Sometimes he is a salesman, with slicked back hair, the fresh citrus smell of Old Spice aftershave masking his morning cigarette as he squeezes his thin black socks over the wire coat hangers he has moulded into sausage shapes, and lays them on the old green enamel Kookaburra wood fire stove to dry.

But to Mum he's just a fool.

"He can never stick at anything. He always thinks he knows better than the boss," she says, her mouth grim. He's also "uncouth", which means he has no manners.

"He's like a horse that's been let out of the stable," she says, as he ambles down the hallway in his singlet and blue shorts, farting noisily, and disappears outside to the toilet, where he keeps his stack of Popular Mechanics, his favourite magazine.

Inspired, he sketches plans on the cream laminate top of our kitchen table with the mechanical pencil he keeps in his top pocket and which never needs sharpening. His hands like all the Cafarellas, are long-fingered and finely boned, with fine blue veins forming rivers and tributaries across his smooth brown skin. His bare brown legs are splayed, and his bare feet in worn rubber thongs, reveal his "hammer toes" – the little toe crossed over the fourth, as if hammered on. Every now and again, he stops sketching and cuts thick slabs of butter, which he plasters on his favourite square Uneeda biscuits, slurping noisily as he dips them in his tea, where the butter forms oily pools.

"How to mould character into drab walls," advises Popular Mechanics, and egged on by Mum, Dad replaces the wall between our dining room and lounge room with an archway covered in thick swirls of white paint, Spanish style. Dad is going to make us a steel-framed garage too, but as winter approaches, the concrete slab fills with puddles and the four fat poles he plants at the corners become thick with orange rust, matching Mum's orange mohair cardigan, which like all our clothes, comes from the SOS op shop.

When our friend Nita Lund complains she is too old and puffed to walk the length of the golf course, Dad sketches plans for a golf buggy and soon fashions a chair from sheet metal, with a square orange plastic cushion that slots neatly into the space he has cut for it. The golf buggy is powered by a two-stroke engine with a joystick to steer it. Julie sits on Dad's knee and I stand on the platform at the back where Nita Lund will put her golf clubs, and we chug along to Nanny's house in Florence Street. Sometimes Julie and I take the golf buggy out on our own, until one day it topples over and burns Julie's shoulder and Mum bans us. When it's finished, Dad sprays it mint green, to contrast with the orange cushion, but Nita Lund never uses it. It's too noisy.

It's Mum who makes us a desk from an old door she paints sky blue and rests on two towers of old bricks, where we sit cutting pictures from magazines and pasting them in our scrap books. On wet days, she lines the wide hallway with her cake tins and baking trays, and the metallic pings turn to soft plops as the tins fill up.

"I'm sick of living off the smell of an oily rag surrounded by crap," she says gazing through the kitchen window at our back yard with its mass of weeds that reach out to choke the few shrubs that dare to survive. Giant wooden cable reels serve as tables, but we don't sit there. The yard is too littered with old car parts, chicken wire, hessian bags, and bits of wood with nails sticking up that twice result in tetanus injections for me.

On a good day she calls him "the pot and pan", rhyming slang for "the old man", and he calls her "wifey", and he nips into the kitchen to whip up a cake for friends – a hangover from his days as an apprentice pastry cook – serving it with ambrosial charm.

On a good day, they play and sing together.

"Bring the guitar," friends plead and Dad throws it in the back of his car with its mess of tools. Dad sings harmony to her melody, in songs that seem to parallel their lives – *The Sweetheart Tree*, about the tree that bursts into bloom when true lovers carve their name in it, *Lemon Tree*, when love turns sour, and *Single Girl* – about the mother who rocks the cradle and cries for the days when she was single and free.

Singing is both a blessing and a curse in our family. Everybody does it – except Mum's sister Doris, whom we call Dottie. Nana Cafarella's mother even died of it after a jealous woman cast the evil eye on her, leaving Nana motherless at just 14 months of age. But nobody can sing like Mum.

My mother's voice is the soundtrack of my childhood. A beautiful effortless soprano, it soars over the clash of dishes, the hum of vacuum cleaners and the relentless pleading of "But Frank ..." as my father flees her scalding tongue.

She spurns the school mothers' club and the fundraising white elephant and cake stalls. Instead, she holds a musical evening at our house in Remo Street, with herself in the starring role of Madam Butterfly, complete with kimono and white face make-up, a rosebud of lipstick centred on her full lips and two knitting needles poking out at right angles from her cobwebby "comb-up".

"The cars were parked all down the street," she says.

She forms a little performing group with two friends. Mum sings all the big numbers – *Velia, the Witch of the Wood,* from The Merry Widow, *This is My Beloved,* from Kismet and Gounod's (and only Gounod's) *Ave Maria*. For comic relief, she sings *Big Spender,* and *Second Hand Rose,* finishing with a duet of *Wish Me Luck As You Wave Me Goodbye*.

There is never enough of this singing for Julie and me. We crave it like sugar and can repeat all the words of the songs like prayers. Once, when Nanny takes us to visit her older brother Uncle Tom, we entertain them, piping away in imitation of our parents, enjoying the way our voices blend. We sing melody, but just like Mum and Dad we are in perfect harmony.

But not for long. On a bad day, he calls her "face-ache" and she calls him "a fool" and "a no-hoper". On the worst days, she follows him from room to room, pleading "But Frank …" as he flees her accusations about the neglected house and the neglected bills, slamming every door in her face until the final slamming of the car door, as he roars off to his friend Jeff or to his big sister Aunty Mary, who calls him "Poor Frankie", for having a wife as useless and unsympathetic as my mother. Sometimes he takes my sister Julie with him.

I follow my mother to the red phone box at the end of the street, where I sit underneath the tall bench, while she talks in a low urgent voice to Nanny or her sister Doris, until there is an impatient rap on the glass, and she says, "I have to go. Someone wants the phone."

"And another thing," Mum says as soon as Dad returns with Julie. And another and another, until he flees again, or on Sundays, retreats to the lounge room to watch "the fight of the century" on World Championship Wrestling, where compere Jack Little tells him in a gravelly Southern drawl, "Neither one will give an inch."

I am glad to be the child of my mother, who is often sick and depends on me, just as I depend on her. "Hold this," she says, as she stands in the bath unravelling oatmeal-coloured crepe bandages from her legs, and the blood trickles from the cuts where her "very close veins" – as Dad calls them – have been stripped. I want to kiss her to make it better. That's my job. I can't recall when I learned this. Just like the story of the half-severed finger, the story she tells me becomes the template for our relationship.

She and Dad were arguing and he hit her, although I could never imagine this. He was always running away, not putting up a fight. It doesn't matter. The point of the story isn't that she suffered, but that I saved her.

"You put your hand in mine, and I thought she understands," she repeats over the years. All I understand is that she is sick and unhappy.

Over the 20 years of her marriage, various bits of her are repaired or removed: her "very close" veins, the pus-filled whitlows and carbuncles on her fingers, her poisoned appendix, the gall bladder full of black stones, her fibroid-ridden womb and the choking goitre visible in the only photo of us all together when I am a baby. They cut it out, leaving a necklace of angry, red, raised scar tissue, which she explained away to strangers by saying she'd left her beads on while sunbaking. Each time she is struck down, I am marooned.

I am seven when she scalds her feet carrying boiling water from the old copper boiler to the big concrete trough in our outside laundry. That night she is hosting Nanny's 70th birthday, so she puts on a pair of Dad's thick black work socks and carries on. By morning, her feet have blown up like pink and peeling party balloons.

"Hurry up," Dad says, as I linger at the foot of the bed where she lies, her mummified feet resting on a pillow. I don't want to go to school without saying goodbye.

"Hurry UP," Dad repeats, frowning. At school, I throw the smelly sardine sandwich he has made for my lunch in the bin.

As I grow older, she asks my advice. What should she say? What should she do about the man and the life and the problems she is tethered to? And like a junior soothsayer, I cast around for solutions. Something. Anything. And somehow the words come. He is wrong. She is right. Everything will be all right – until she claps her hands with relief and delight, exclaiming: "You've hit the nail on the head!" leaving me feeling powerful and guilty, fearful of what she will do with these words.

I never tell Julie what Mum and I say and do together when we are alone, and she never tells me what she and Dad say and do together when he takes her in the car when they fight. We take our positions, like soldiers, armed and unquestioning.

"She threw the banana sandwich at the teacher," Mum says when we are alone, telling me again how we missed out on kindergarten because Julie refused to be bribed into attendance. We didn't go to the book parade at school either, as Julie refused to enter the school grounds because someone was dressed as a witch, even though Mum had made her a Bo Peep outfit of blue crepe paper, complete with bonnet, crook and a lamb, cut out of cardboard and covered in cotton balls. At Christmas, as we sit on Santa's knee for a photo, Julie sticks out her bottom jaw and pulls a face.

Mum and Julie don't love each other, but they both love animals. Mum was a country girl, wild and plain, born in Wycheproof, in Victoria, catching yabbies and riding horses with her friend Jimmy Welwood – famously chopping the legs off Pa's best trousers when she couldn't find her jodhpurs. She had a pet Magpie she taught to talk, and a scruffy Airedale dog called Cougar, who used to sing along with the church organist.

A house isn't a home without a dog, Mum says when a friend gives her a pedigree bulldog puppy, called Samantha.

"Let's go and see Sammy," Julie says when we wake early one morning, though Mum has forbidden it. We sneak out to the trailer in the backyard where Sammy is sleeping in a bundle of our old jumpers. Sammy's fur, the colour of blanched almonds, hangs in soft folds around her black squashed-in face, as she snuggles into Julie's chest.

The next week Sammy is dead. Her heart failed under the anaesthetic while she was being spayed. Mum cries for days. She suspects Sammy still lives, secretly coveted by the vet who has lied to us so he can claim her. Dad rushes out to buy a consoling present, returning with a pink tin of biscuits with adorable Labrador puppies on the lid, which sets Mum crying anew. Soon after, Sammy is replaced by a small brown mongrel called Lizzie, named after Queen Elizabeth because she was the boss of her litter. Lizzie is so smart Mum only has to say "Let's go to the beach", or "Let's go to the shops", and Lizzie heads in the right direction.

I love Lizzie, but not as much as Mum and Julie do. I'm not sure if I love Julie, who throws hot water over me in the bath, and talc in my eyes when Mum isn't looking. The water isn't that hot, and doesn't burn, and the talc mostly misses, so I don't tell. Nor do I tell when Julie scrapes the toes of her new school shoes on the gravel on the way home from school to ruin them when Mum refuses to buy the more fashionable pointy-toed shoes, which are no good for school. I feel sorry for Mum who doesn't have any more money for shoes.

Sisters are not to be trusted. Like Dad's big sister Aunty Mary, who is like Julie – perverse.

"I came back from going to the toilet one day and she was going through my purse," Mum says, wide-eyed.

Mum's big sister, Dottie is perverse too. "She used to pinch and twist the flesh on my arm when we were children, and make me get out of bed to turn out the light, even though she knew I was scared of the dark," Mum tells me.

Yet on Christmas Day, we eat roast chicken and plum pudding at Dottie's big red brick house in Union Road, Balwyn, arriving at the Cafarella Christmas late in the day when all the adults are sleeping off the polpetta, cotoletta and cannoli and our cousins, with their concertos of Italian names, are running wild.

"Look out for the blue bus," Mum says, when Dad is at work at weekends, as we wait at Mentone station for the blue Ventura bus that will hiss and groan all the way down Warrigal Road to Union Road, to Dottie's house in Balwyn, to see our other cousins, Joel, Pip and Pam – and where Nanny calls me "darkie" and my cousins call me "Janey" or "Janey Lou" or "Lulu Belle".

Dottie is "comfortable", which means debt collectors never come to her door and she doesn't have to put all her cake tins down the hallway when it rains. Aunty Iris, their cousin, who lives on an orchard in Doncaster, is also comfortable. Every month, Dottie, Aunty Iris and Mum meet at the fashionable Café Vienna at the Australia Hotel for lunch, which makes Mum extremely uncomfortable as she has no money and nothing to wear.

Dottie's husband has a "good position" with a big company, a job he has stuck at for as long as anyone can remember. His name is John, but in our infant babble Julie and I call him Da, which sticks.

"Can we have a whizzy?" Julie and I plead, as Da sweeps us up in his arms when we visit. Julie goes first. Da holds her firmly by one arm and one leg and whizzes her around in wide circles, until she squeals with terror and delight. Then it's my turn. Da holds me by my left arm and my good left leg and the world whizzes past.

Dottie and Da never ask about my leg. No one does, not even Mum or Dad. Nor do I expect them to. But at school the other children point, whisper, stare and chant, "You've got one fat and one skinny leg."

"Tell them you were born that way, and nothing can be done about it," Mum says, which mostly shuts them up. Julie and I don't play together at school, as we are in different classes. I befriend a girl call Susan, who has one hand permanently closed in a claw, the palm a patchwork of scar tissue. Susan wasn't born that way. She was three when her big brother dared her to grasp the red-hot bar of the exposed radiator.

At bedtime I close my eyes and begin a new game, which is to think of the best thing that happened to me that day and the best thing that will happen to me the next day. "Oh ho my nut brown maiden," Mum sings when she comes to kiss me good night, followed by my favourite … "Here we go, in a golden boat, far away, far away," and together we float far away from the teasing and the fighting.

2

For a while, Mum fears I might be perverse too.

"Pay attention," she says, thumping me between my shoulder blades when I stare at the clouds as we walk home from Nanny's one afternoon.

I didn't know I wasn't.

"She's ignoring me," she tells Dad over dinner, and he ignores us both.

Months later I find myself sitting across from a man in a white coat, who studies me with his sad brown eyes. Mum tells him about my "turns" and I have a turn right in front of him. My head is x-rayed and I am taken to a small room where a nurse puts sticky cream in my hair and a rubber cap on my head. The cap is connected with wires to a machine. "Close your eyes," a nurse instructs. "Open, close, open, close. Good girl."

The doctor tells my mother my head is normal but my brain is not. From then on, after every meal, I chew two square musk-flavoured tablets called Tridione, dispensed from the hospital pharmacy in a big brown glass jar. Mum tells me I have petit mal, meaning "little sickness" which I later learn is a form of childhood epilepsy that causes "absences". The word epilepsy never crosses her lips.

I enjoy taking the day off school to visit the outpatient clinic at the hospital, wearing my best clothes and sipping chilled water from conical paper cups dispensed from a machine in the waiting room.

"How are you?" asks the kind doctor with the sad eyes, whose name is Dr Coldbeck. I smile and say, "Very well, thank you."

"She's doing very well at school," Mum says, and I beam, even though when I first start school I do "mirror writing", writing every letter backwards.

"And how's the leg?" Dr Coldbeck asks.

"The same," Mum says, and they exchange knowing looks about the problem that has no name and for which there is no cure.

Afterwards, Mum rewards me with a steaming hot meat pie and a pink and frothy strawberry milkshake from the hospital canteen.

Once or twice at home, I smell something purple and fall to the ground. Mum's voice calls from far away. "Jane! Jane! Wake up!" But I don't want to wake up. I am busy in my dream. Her voice grows louder as I come to the surface and vomit into the towel she holds.

"You've had a turn," she says, and I shiver and shake in bed for the rest of the day.

On summer nights, she pushes my bed against the wall and places all our kitchen chairs around it, in case I have a turn in the night and fall out. I don't know where Julie is while I am in bed shivering. We never talk together about my visits to Dr Coldbeck or my turns. She only goes to the hospital once, when she climbs the forbidden scaffolding at the house next door and falls off, breaking her arm.

Mum had elocution lessons as child – "I had such a plum in my mouth people used to stare at me," she says – which qualifies her to treat my other problem.

"Say snake," she says, as she rubs me dry with a thin towel that has graduated from beach towel to bath towel.

"Shhhhnake."

"No. SSSSSSnake," she says, night after night until one night I say, "Snake!"

"She's got it! She's got it!" Mum cries.

"She's very well adjusted," she tells family and friends who inquire about my new affliction. She doesn't tell them about the mural of green snot – or "goosh" as I call it – that I create on the wall beside my bed. Strangely, this habit goes unnoticed, until one summer night when the light cast by a dazzling sunset illuminates my goosh mural.

"What's this?" Mum says, after she kisses me goodnight, her green goosh-coloured eyes widening as she leans across the chairs around my bed.

"Goosh," I say softly, clutching the quilt to my chin, my heart suspended in my chest like a bell mid-gong.

"Goosh?"

I translate. "Shnot."

The next day reconstituted snot trickles down the wall as, shamefaced, I dip a rag in a bucket of warm grey water to remove it. I give up nose picking and replace it with teeth grinding, discovered when Mum hears squeaking as she passes my room. There is no treatment for this, so it's ignored. Chewing follows grinding.

"She ate the hair right off it!" Mum tells visitors, pointing to the spikey Frankenstein-like scalp of the walking doll she saved up for. I burn with embarrassment – especially as Julie's walking doll still has a full head of rich brown nylon curls.

The Tridione tablets make me prone to "bilious attacks", which means I throw up a lot. Being sick becomes normal, but I am not sickly. I am sturdy, with a rather too healthy appetite, which delights Mum, as Julie is a "fussy eater".

"You followed the spoon," Mum tells me gleefully, her mouth agape in imitation of my infant self, waiting to be filled up.

Dad is less impressed. "God, Jane's a dead weight," he says when Mum tells him to piggy back me over some slippery rocks at a family excursion, while later, at home, Julie sits lightly on his knee.

While I am being filled up, my sister is … I don't know. I am in a fog as my body adjusts to the tablets. When the fog lifts, Julie and I play together with the kids who live at the gasworks across the road, climbing on the big green-painted pipes and rolling down the hills until our jumpers are prickly with burrs. In the May and September school holidays we go to Aunty Iris's orchard in Doncaster, to play with our cousin Julianna, who has the name my sister was supposed to have – except Aunty Iris spells it with two ns.

At Aunty Iris's we are *The Three Jays*, Julianna, Julie and Jane. We roam the orchard, perfumed with the scent of apples and pears, and watch the men in the packing shed in their thick leather aprons, cradling brown pears in blankets of tissue paper and tucking them into boxes, while Julianna's snowy-haired brother Nicholas rides his tricycle around and around the dusty floorboards.

At Aunty Iris's, flagons of Doncaster Apple Juice squat on the table during Sunday lunch, and crates of Loy's soft drink in every flavour are delivered every month, even when it's nobody's birthday. At night as we watch television, Aunty Iris strokes our hair and calls us "Floss", and every day she makes morning and afternoon tea for Uncle Pete, who comes in from the orchard wearing faded blue overalls and a gentle smile.

At Aunty Iris's there are no fights. In Remo Street, there are so many that Dad is moving out for a "trial separation". I don't know where he goes, maybe to Aunty Mary's.

On weekends he returns with small bits of bloody newspaper stuck to his chin and takes Julie and me to the movies. We see *Born Free* three times, embedding the title song in my memory.

Easter Bunny, whom we know is Mum, leaves us one big egg each and two small ones. Dad brings us each a boxed Red Tulip set with one big egg in the middle, circled by foil-covered chocolates, pink for me and gold for Julie. We tally our treasure – 16 eggs each, counting the chocolates. Dad wins.

Then Dad comes back and sings *The Green Green Grass of Home*, and it's the "wifey" and the "pot and pan" again, until one day a big board goes up outside our house telling everyone our life is for sale.

3

Our new home is a two-bedroom flat just around the corner in Patty Street, Mentone near the railway line, where we move with one dog and two mice while we wait for our brand new A.V. Jennings house in the brand-new suburb of Mulgrave to be built, and where Dad is a Jennings salesman. It takes a whole year of visiting display homes for Mum and Dad to decide on the design – a double-fronted chocolate brick veneer called The Ashley.

By the time our new house is ready a year later, we have nine dogs and 40 mice, the result of Lizzie's late-night liaison with a local mutt and the surprising fact that our sister mice turned out to be husband and wife.

"Can we keep a puppy?" pleads Julie, but Mum says one dog is enough, and she gives all the puppies and mice away, and then wishes she hadn't when Lizzie is run over and has to be "put down". Moving to the new house in Redfern Crescent Mulgrave feels less exciting without Lizzie.

"We'll get a new dog for the new house," Dad promises.

The only piece of furniture from our past life to cross the threshold of The Ashley is our piano. Everything else is too big. Dad builds a small table in the kitchen, hinged to the wall so it can be folded away. The idea so appeals to him that he builds our television into the corner of our new lounge room, with the screen hinged to the side for easy access to its multicoloured intestines during its many breakdowns. The TV repairman's mouth swings open in a similar fashion every time he comes to fix it.

As a housewarming present, Dad brings home a small black puppy with a white muzzle, whom he names Mini Moke, after a type of car. Mini isn't as smart as Lizzie, but we love her all the same.

A housewarming present arrives from Dottie and Aunty Iris – two glass chandeliers with garlands of crystal teardrops – just like the chandeliers in their houses, except slung from The Ashley's low ceilings, they seem to highlight the smallness of the lounge room, making all the big dreams of our parents seem small.

Nanny, Dottie and Aunty Iris don't visit and we don't visit them either as, at first, Mum doesn't have a car and there is no train, just infrequent buses. We are so busy fixing up The Ashley we don't have time to miss them. Dad borrows Aunty Mary's sewing machine and makes pinch-pleat curtains from thick pavlova-coloured fibre-glass material, and the neighbours watch gobsmacked as with a few cactus plants, pebbles, black plastic and grey, open "Besser" bricks, in one afternoon Mum and Dad create what the Japanese took centuries to perfect – a "Japanese" rock garden. We meet the neighbours when they come running with buckets after Dad lights our incinerator on a hot windy day and our fence catches fire.

At our new school, where I am in Grade Four and Julie is in Grade Five, freckle-faced Michael tells me what I already know – "You've got one fat and one skinny leg."

Michael has curly ginger hair, a nose like a pig, and so many orange freckles on his pale round face he looks like someone spat tea all over it. I guess he was born that way. To shut him up, I kick him in the shins with my good leg. That night I tell Mum I kicked him with my *hind* leg, which sends her into hysterics. Kicking Michael shows I am "well-adjusted", which means not giving in.

Julie learns that she, too, is imperfect. "Witchipoo!" the kids taunt, naming her after the witch in the new television series Adventure

Island, because like everyone in our family she has a big nose. I'm used to being different, but Julie is upset.

"Just ignore them," Mum says.

We are both relieved when the school is declared too big and we are syphoned off to a new school called Wellington Primary, where I am a library monitor, helping cover the new books in clear plastic, and Julie is so good at high jump that Dad makes a special high jump for the school, with shiny black tape wound in a candy stripe around the white poles. I try too, but my real passion is getting 10 out of 10 for everything, because when I get nine, Dad says, "What happened to the other mark?"

I am 12, standing by the laundry trough bathing Mini and talking to Mum when I smell something purple again and fall down. It's the second turn I've had in just a few months. If I have any more, Dr Coldbeck says I'll have to go off Tridione, and go on a drug called phenobarbital. A turn like that means we can't have two-wheeler bikes, in case I black out in the middle of the road, and because what Mum "does for one she does for the other".

I don't care. While Julie watches *Uptight* on television, dancing along to the latest pop songs, and reads *Dolly* magazine to find out what to wear and what to say to boys, my friend Alison and I play with our Pee Wee dolls, making dolls houses from cardboard boxes with matchbox furniture. On a big sheet of poster paper, I map out a world for them named Palicia – like a palace – illustrated with texta pens and water colours.

"Look what Jane drew," Mum says, showing everyone, and with the money she earns at the Wanda Street Milk Bar, she buys me oil paints and an easel. She is thrilled with my muddy purple painting of amorphous figures sitting around wine barrels, after a rare family excursion to Frank Traynor's folk club in the city.

"What God takes with one hand, he gives with the other," she says – meaning God has compensated for my asymmetrical brain and legs by giving me artistic TALENT, which it is her job to ENCOURAGE.

For a while, she thinks I might have singing talent, too. I stand stiffly by our piano, my eyes popping as I try to scale the mountainous high notes while Mum plods through *Feed the Birds* from Mary Poppins. I am scared of repeating the failure of *The Ugly Duckling*, which I sang for Nana Cafarella when I was seven and which Mum said I'd sung "through my nose".

But at Redfern Crescent, Mum is always ENCOURAGING.

"Will I have a voice as good as you?" I ask.

"Better," she says, and we both know she is lying.

The quest for talent is unrelenting. While Dad works nightshift at a factory and Julie stays in her room reading about pop stars in *TV Week*, Mum and I watch *New Faces* hosted by Frank Wilson, and *Showcase*, hosted by Gordon Boyd with the Hector Crawford Orchestra, where contestants compete to be "discovered".

Showcase is our favourite. I sit in my pyjamas next to Mum, who holds a glass of sherry in her left hand and a Benson and Hedges in her right. Her head is cocked, listening, her gaze on the young contestant, who is singing sweetly. Silently, Mum mouths the words of the song as it should be sung. She sighs and taps her cigarette on the burnt-orange coloured pottery ashtray before delivering her verdict.

"A soubrette," she says, dismissively.

I don't know what a soubrette is but I know from the contempt in my mother's voice that this is something she would never be. The girl doesn't win. I knew she wouldn't. Mum is seldom wrong when it comes to assessing talent. The contestants that follow are all bad. Their diction is bad, their intonation is bad, their "head voices" need work, they dress badly, they need to stand up straight and breathe from their diaphragms, which is somewhere near your stomach because that's where Mum presses when she says the word. Mum breathes from her diaphragm even when she's under anaesthetic, as the doctors always ask her afterwards, "Are you a singer?"

Only sometimes does she pronounce, "She's good." The good ones have TALENT. No one is good on New Faces, where people forget the words.

After school, Mum leans over the piano helping me work out the notes as I plod through *Greensleeves*. Sometimes, she teaches me vaudeville songs from The Tivoli Theatre, like *Little Sir Echo*, with its chorus of echoing hellos. Sometimes, we play an echoing game.

"Baaa …" Mum says, bleating like a goat, daring me to follow.

"Baaaa," I reply. On and on, baaa, baaa, baaa, laughing at the absurdity of it, until Dad yells at us to shut up.

Whenever she can afford it, Mum buys us books about adventurous girls, like *Heidi* and Katy in *What Katy Did*.

"Just one more chapter," I beg, when she comes to kiss me good night, singing "Oh ho, my nut brown maiden," followed by "Sweet dreams! Sleep tight! Hope the bed bugs don't bite."

I'm up to the part where Katy is crippled and angry after falling off a swing, until her angelic invalid Cousin Helen tells her everyone has a rough handle and a smooth handle and life is much better if you choose the smooth handle.

After school, Julie begs Mum to buy her witches britches: frilly nylon shorts worn by all the Grade Six girls under their school dresses to hide their knickers when their dresses blow up in the wind. Mum doesn't trust them, just as she doesn't trust the new craze for pantyhose, which don't allow girls to breathe "down there". She buys us suspender belts and stockings, which Julie flatly refuses to wear.

"She's wearing her mother's suspenders," a girl shrieks when the wind blows my dress up during a game of elastics, revealing one stocking stretched sheer over my big leg while the other stocking remains opaque, and so Mum relents and buys me pantyhose too.

The following year, Julie starts high school and has her first period. Dad has a new job selling welding rods for a company called Eutectic and is away. Julie sits on the toilet with the door open, talking to Mum, who has just taught her how to put on a Modess belt, a thin elastic belt that fits around her waist to hold the pad between her legs.

"My stomach hurts," Julie says.

"That's normal," Mum says and she brings her some Aspirin and says it will go away soon.

I stand at the bathroom door, naked under my dressing gown, delaying my shower, enjoying this women's talk, which feels strangely companionable.

Mum turns her focus to me. "Let's see how you're developing."

I freeze. I am 13 and perfectly aware of how I'm developing: hair sprouting inconveniently under my arms, swelling breasts and nipples that have expanded from brown buttons to plump raspberries. My leg is developing, too. My right buttock is bigger and rounder than the left and everything "down there" is swollen. I don't want to show Mum. I don't want to show anyone. But I have no words to say how I feel, so slowly, silently, I remove my dressing gown and stand flushed and naked, trying to focus on my long brown arms with the fine muscle definition I have inherited from Dad.

Mum walks around me, inspecting me from every angle. "You're developing well," she says, as if I've passed a test.

Part of me knows her true motive. She's assessing the damage. How big is my "big leg" now – and what to do about it? Although we all know nothing can be done. From the corner of my eye, I feel Julie's sharp-eyed disgust as she watches this play-acting. It's plain weird and we both know it, although we never discuss it.

Soon after, the books Mum gives me change from the stories of adventurous girls like Katy to stories about people triumphing over adversity, like *I Can Jump Puddles,* by Alan Marshall and *My Life* by Helen Keller. Helen Keller is an insufferable saint but I love Alan Marshall, who jumps puddles and rides horses even though he can't walk, and who notices what people say and how they say it, like me.

"Why don't you write to him?" Mum says, and she helps me find his address. To my surprise he writes back in his own handwriting, which I'd insisted upon. Anyone could type a letter: handwriting made it real. I am disappointed to hear I am one of many children who write to him, but he promises we will be pen pals, although from now on, his secretary Gwen will type his letters.

"What do you look like?" I ask.

"I am a short plain unattractive man, as bald as an egg," he replies. It's not until my third letter that I tell him how I look.

"It delights me to know that one of your legs is larger than the other," he replies. "I would have you no other way. In my experience a person with a handicap always compensates by developing charm and personality, which I'm sure you have in abundance."

I don't, but I plan to in future.

The following year I start high school. "What do we have next?" I ask the girl next to me as we pull books from grey metal lockers for the next period. What's next is my first period, which comes in an embarrassing flood. The two pads Mum has tucked into my school bag aren't enough, and I'm given permission to go to a friend's place, which is closer, where we raid the neatly arranged pads in the bottom drawer in her mother's bedroom. It doesn't occur to me to ask Julie for help. Our paths seldom cross at school. At home, we are like two characters in the same play who seldom share a scene together. Once when I am cross with her, I draw a moustache on one of her favourite pop stars. She retaliates by drawing a moustache on my postcard of a bird.

Dad is working at Repco, as a salesman, and buys us bikes, which is now allowed, as my turns have almost gone away. But Julie is more interested in fashion.

"I want to be a model," she says at the dinner table one night, and complains she has no calf muscles. Dad says she's mispronounced it: what she'll really be is a "muddle".

"There's nothing wrong with her legs," Mum snaps when Dad's younger sister Tess visits and shows her some exercises to improve her calf muscles on her two identical legs.

"Can I go to The Swan?" Julie says, one night over dinner, looking at Mum.

"What's the Swan?" Mum says.

"A billiard parlour. All the kids go there."

"You're not going there."

Billiard parlours are full of shady men. No place for young girls, Mum says.

"Let her go," Dad says.

Mum shoots him the same disapproving look she gives Julie.

"You're not going."

"It's not fair," Julie says, flouncing to her room.

"Don't answer back," Mum says.

I sit in my room at my desk with the map of the world top, copying a map of Thailand for an assignment, glad to be the good girl who never causes trouble.

A few months later, Julie turns 14 and invites her new best friend Valerie to our family celebration. Valerie is of West Indian descent with dark wavy hair, an oval face and golden skin, and who is so pretty that every other girl squirms in her presence. But to Mum, she's just a girl with no manners.

"She didn't even bring a present," Mum whispers to me.

Julie doesn't seem to notice. She and Valerie sit at the kitchen table laughing and joking about things I don't understand, which makes them laugh and joke more.

"You're a dag," Julie tells me. She glances at Valerie for approval, who smiles her beautiful smile.

"I bet you don't even know what that means," Julie says, regarding me with narrowed eyes.

I do, and am keen to prove it.

"A dag is a piece of pooh," I say primly.

Julie and Valerie laugh their heads off, because I have just proved them right.

Mum and Julie fight about Valerie, and Julie's other friends, who are The Wrong Company. They all speak badly. They are common – and A Bad Influence. "Why can't you find some nice friends, like Jane's?"

Julie wants to wear her dresses short. Mum says no. Julie wants to wear make-up. Mum says no.

"Leave her alone," Dad says.

"You don't care what she does or who she's with, but I do," Mum yells, and she tells Julie she is "round shouldered" and to stand up straight and speak properly.

"It's not fair!" Julie says.

"She's a pill, isn't she? Why is she like this?" Mum says, answering her own question with the familiar refrain: "The apple doesn't fall far from the tree." And the tree says leave her alone, let her go, let her fall.

As she falls, I rise. During the week, Mum helps me with my school projects. Our Form One class is part of an experiment called Integrated Studies, the brainchild of Bryan, our neighbour, who teaches at the high school. The only subjects we study formally are Indonesian and Maths. The rest we can explore in more creative and integrated ways, through paintings, plays or presentations. The end of the month is Show Time. Mum buys hessian and dowel and coloured wool for a wall hanging I design of a fish in the ocean, and bake-at home clay in red and grey for the chess set I create on a small table that I tile under her tuition in matching red and grey.

"Look at Jane, be like Jane," she tells Julie.

But the clay is too heavy and the King and Queen list dangerously to the side, their crowned heads sinking into their shoulders, defeated. I am defeated too. There are too many assignments. When my friend Alison comes over to play, I send her away. I'm in high school now. Most nights I sit in my room working until two in the morning, only stopping when I hear the key in the door as Dad returns from night shift, followed by his snores when he falls asleep in the bath.

"Dad, Dad! Wake up," I call through the bathroom door, fearing he'll drown, and the swish of water tells me he's heard me.

Julie's problems happen outside of this, a distant thunder. I don't realise there is a storm brewing until one shimmery hot summer morning before school, when she stops me in the driveway.

"What time does Mum get home from work?"

It's a request for information, not a conversation.

"About four," I say. "Why?"
"Just asking," she says, and walks ahead to the bus stop.
That night she doesn't come home.

4

Mum's voice rises an octave with each question: "Are you SURE she didn't say where she was going? Did she take any money? Did she say who she was going with? Are you SURE?"

"Yes," I say, dully. "I'm sure."

That night, we wait for the police to call and tell us Julie is at Valerie's place, defiant and cocky, happy to have punished us all so thoroughly.

But there is no call. Nobody knows where she is: not the school, not the neighbours, no one. Teatime becomes bedtime. Through my bedroom wall, I hear Dad's hoarse sobs and Mum's frantic whispers.

"Julie's run away," Mum says when they finally emerge, stunned and scared. The police are searching for her.

"Why has she done this? What's wrong with her?" Mum says.

I know why. It's because of them and because of me, because just like Katy when she falls off the swing and hurts her back in *What Katy Did*, Julie is angry and has life by the rough handle, while I have it by the smooth.

A week goes by. I go to school as normal, but nothing is normal. Mum and Dad make an emotional plea on the radio, "Julie, we love you, please come home."

That night after school, Dad takes me on his knee. "You're all we've got now," he says, and it occurs to me that my sister might be dead: abducted or murdered like the schoolgirls whose pictures appear in the newspapers and who will be schoolgirls forever. A week ago I was a sister. Today I am an only child, sitting lightly on Dad's knee. Perhaps I am glad to be an only child?

As the weeks drag by, Mum and Dad move from fear to blame and back to fear, while the neighbours visit and console, and everyone waits, dreading and willing the phone to ring. "They've found her," Mum says, when it does, and everyone cries. Except me. It's as if I'm standing outside all of this, watching a movie, which I hope will soon be over.

The police found her hitch-hiking back to Melbourne, Mum says. Nobody knew where she slept, or worse still, who with, just that she was alone. Mum and Dad leave immediately for Wagga Wagga in New South Wales, where there will be a court case.

Where do I stay? I don't remember. Maybe with our neighbours across the road? It doesn't matter. I am relieved and guilty for being the good girl with bad thoughts.

Two days later, Mum and Dad return without her. "We're waiting for things to be resolved," Mum says, as we sit with Dad at the kitchen table in Redfern Crescent.

"She told the judge to get fucked," Mum says, shaking her head in disgust, and I am amazed at the cheek of my sister, who answers back to a judge, and that my mother has said "fucked" when I got into trouble for saying "Shitty shitty bang bang".

The judge said Julie was "exposed to moral danger" and was "uncontrollable" but she wasn't charged with anything because she was "a minor", Mum says.

Later, when Dad is at work and we are alone, Mum tells me, "The Judge asked 'Who will take responsibility for this child?' – I was the only one who put up my hand! I was!"

I wonder why Dad, who sobbed when Julie ran away, didn't put up his hand.

If it wasn't for Mum putting up her hand, Julie would have been declared a "ward of the state" and sent to Winlaton, the notorious home for wayward girls. Mum has saved her.

While things are being resolved with Julie, we are going on holiday to a place called Yarrawonga on the Murray River, near the NSW border. Dad shows us a pamphlet. A lake of blue water laps grassy banks. Laughing children swing across it, holding on to a rope called a flying fox. Gleaming caravans with miniature stoves, fridges and beds are shaded by white gums with blue-green leaves. I don't know how we can afford this gleaming holiday or why Julie doesn't come. Perhaps she didn't want to? I don't care. I'm looking forward to a holiday with no arguments, where I am still an only child. But there is no escape.

"She told the judge to get fucked!" Mum repeats as we cross the New South Wales border and I stare through the car window, my legs sticking to the seat.

"Wait here," Dad, says when we finally arrive at the caravan park, and he goes to find the manager. I lean out the window. Brown water laps muddy banks. The playground is old and rusty. The grass is browned off. There are few trees.

"You can go for a swim but be careful of the leeches," Dad says when he returns with the key to our caravan. Leeches are water worms that stick to your skin and suck your blood out, Mum explains.

"Where's the flying fox?" I ask Dad.

"Out of order."

While Mum unpacks tins of soup and milk and bread, I change into my bathers and jeans and go down to the jetty. I'm glad there's no one there. The stiff conical bra cups of my bright yellow and orange one-piece bathers stand erect even when I lay down to sunbake, promising something I can't deliver. I sit on the edge of the jetty, anxious and upright, peering into the milky brown water, searching for leeches.

"Hi," a voice behind me says. A boy of about 16, with a round brown face and brown straight hair smiles down at my conical bosom. His name is Michael Moon and his family own a sheep station further north.

"Do you want to come water skiing tomorrow?"

"No, thank you."

All I know about water skiing is that you need two feet the same.

"Come for a swim, then," he says, and I'm surprised when Mum says I can go.

The next morning, my stomach jolts as the boat slaps hard against the water as Michael's ruddy father steers it into the middle of the lake, which is clear and blue and leech free.

"Come on!" Michael says, and he dives in, laughing and shaking his hair like a wet happy dog as he surfaces. I wait till he looks the other way before removing my t-shirt and jeans and lowering myself into the water via a metal ladder at the side of the boat. The water envelops me. Yarrawonga is improving.

Late that night, as I lay in the narrow top bunk, a sharp rap rattles the caravan door. Dad answers.

"It's the police. We have to go home," he says.

The police say Julie has broken into our house in Redfern Crescent, or another house. I'm never sure which.

"Why is she like this? What's wrong with her?" Mum says, as we leave Yarrawonga and Michael Moon behind.

5

The tantalising smell of freshly roasted chicken wafts from its foil shroud beneath a tea towel in the picnic basket on the flat bluestone sea wall. Carefully, Mum pours orange juice into the paper cups lined up next to it: one for Dad, one for me, and one for Julie.

I haven't seen her for two months – not since the morning in early December when she asked me what time Mum came home from work. Across the road, behind a long concrete wall is her new home – The Convent of the Good Shepherd – where she is working in the laundry until correspondence school starts.

I don't know how this was decided, just that two weeks earlier on another Sunday, Mum tells me to wait in the convent dining room while she and Dad follow a nun with a face like an elderly cherub down a long corridor. An hour later, they emerge with the nun, who clasps Mum's hands and tells her everything will be all right. God will see to it.

This Sunday is "parlour" – visiting day. We have special permission to be leaning against the sea wall, with our cups of orange juice, and all Julie's favourite foods in the picnic basket, the distant screech of seagulls muted by the gentle lap of the waves and the chatter of children playing.

Julie answers Mum's questions about school in staccato monosyllables: "Yes. No. Leave me alone."

She doesn't look at me.

I sip my orange juice, aware of our changed status: prisoner and free. I hope Mum doesn't tell her about my school report card, declaring in neat black calligraphy that I'm the second Dux of the school, with 16 As.

Julie doesn't drink her orange juice. She turns to me. Perhaps she knows? What do I say to her? Something stupid? Nothing at all? It doesn't matter. With a flick of her wrist, she flings the orange juice in my face. The picnic ends abruptly, confirming Mum's view that they have "done the right thing".

On the way home, Mum tells me we are moving and I will have a new home and school too.

"Your father's gone bankrupt again," she says, staring ahead, her eyes dry and her face like a slammed door.

* * *

The house in Redfern Crescent still hasn't sold but for some reason we've moved to a two-bedroom flat in Alfred Street in Highett, near Southland, until Dad finds us a house. My new school is in Moorabbin, not far from our old stomping ground in Mentone.

"Come on, Jane," the teacher says, cajoling me to try harder, as my classmates sidestep doing "the stomp" to the Daddy Cool song *Eagle Rock* in front of me. Inside I feel like a weary old soldier who's been inadvertently plucked from a war zone and dropped in a class of effervescent and carefree adolescents. Smiling is only possible through an act of will, despite Alan's advice to have "charm and personality in abundance".

The flat is temporary, the school is temporary and my new friend Kerry, who invites me to a local square dance is temporary. I can't dance, but I am desperate to get away from Mum and Dad who glower at each other every night across the dinner table. Kerry doesn't know I'm not a real friend, just someone saying my lines in a show that I desperately want to end.

Then one day it does.

"Papillomas," the local doctor says, when Mum takes me to find out why the sole of my big foot is like a pink ham dotted with black cloves. The doctor sticks a needle into the biggest one and I scream, which brings Mum running.

"Don't you touch her," she yells, and in desperation she calls the Children's Hospital. I am slowly being weaned off Tridione, the petit mal drug, and am technically too old to be a new patient with a new problem. But Mum pleads my case and once again we catch the tram down Flemington Road to the hospital each week, where a matronly doctor dabs each black dot with a freezing liquid so she can dig them out, creating a landscape of miniature craters. At the same time, a visit to the dentist reveals my shameful habit of grinding Arnott's Assorted Cream biscuits to dust while doing my homework. I need 14 fillings, one for every year of my life.

"You've been topped and tailed," Mum says, as we trudge between the dentist and the hospital, while I worry about how we'll pay for all these medical expenses.

"Waiting for a letter from your boyfriend?" Dad says, making me blush when I inspect the letterbox in our new flat in Alfred Street yet again for a letter from Alan Marshall – my only solace. A bald 74-year-old man feels like the only boyfriend I'm likely to get, as angry pink pimples have formed across my forehead and chin, made worse when I have my period, when my hair hangs in oily strands as Mum won't let me wash it.

Letters from Julie in the convent come every few days and Mum is busy buying all the things she asks for – pantyhose, pens, paper and Physohex ointment to dry up the pimples on her back. I have to wait weeks, sometimes months, for a letter from Alan, as he has many children to write to.

When he does write, it's about books and life in the bush, assuming that like him, I'm only temporarily enduring city life. I tell him I want to be a journalist, and perhaps even a writer, and he tells me to read a book about wizards called *The Lord of the Rings*.

I don't tell him about Julie, the fillings or the papillomas when Mum and Dad take me to meet him in his home in Black Rock, where he lives with his sister Elsie. A week later, he writes to me about our "happy visit", predicting I'll have a future in writing "or some other kindred operation".

He has believed that version of myself, that version of our family. He doesn't know our house is gone, Mum is sick with giant fibroids filling her womb and there is no room for more unhappy people in the cramped flat where Julie comes on weekends and where everyone is awkward.

We are all relieved when Dad finally finds us a house in Heslop Street, Parkdale, a short walk from the beach. It's past nine at night, when he takes me to see it. We stand on the veranda in the dark, carrying buckets, mops and bottles of Lysol disinfectant.

"What's that smell?" I say, as the front door swings open.

"The place was owned by an old lady with two retarded daughters," Dad says as he flashes his torch down the dusty corridor. "Sometimes they didn't make it to the toilet."

I don't complain. Julie is in the convent; Mum is in hospital recovering from a hysterectomy. I am all he's got.

"Start in the hallway," Dad says, and together, on our knees, we scrub the dusty boards until the smell goes and the dawn comes.

"Why did he do that?' Mum says, when she finds out. "He should have waited until after settlement."

I'm glad he didn't. Daylight reveals the house has a name: *Wavertree*, stuck on the big concrete veranda in white concrete capitals. It rhymes with lavatory, which seems appropriate, as does the street name – He*SLOP*. The house is a Californian Bungalow, Dad says, but soon it will be a mansion.

The prickly puce-coloured stucco that tries to snare us as we pass will be stripped and repainted gleaming white, and the cavernous sloping roof will house another storey with pretty dormer windows, just like the big white weatherboard house next door. A lift will replace the old wooden linen cupboard in the hallway – but first Dad and I must renovate the fireplace surrounding the rattly old brown gas heater.

"Hand me the trowel," Dad says, as he expertly swishes mortar over the brick surround, while I stand ready to hand him the brown tiles that come in a sheet joined with white mesh. Two days later, he surveys the result.

"It looks like a bloody urinal."

"No, it doesn't," I chirp. I've never seen a urinal anyway.

Our next project is to fix the roof.

"Jane!" he calls as he throws a broken tile, meaning for me to stay out of the way, but I come running and it hits me on the forehead. Dad clamps an oily rag over my forehead and rushes me to the doctor, where I have four stitches and he faints. I cut my hair into fashionable bangs to hide the scar, and start to wash my hair whenever I want to.

On the first day of my new school in Mentone, they stare and ask about my leg and I tell them I'm born that way. I am surprised when a girl who slighted me at primary school approaches me – a bigger version of her former self, except her skirt is so short you can see her knickers when she bends over, and her eyebrows are plucked into tiny stitches.

"Do you have money for the canteen, do you have a boyfriend and do you do it?" she demands.

I lie on all counts. I don't care about the canteen, but I do care about the boyfriend. I don't admit it, even to my diary, but the thing I want most is to wake up one morning with two normal legs and an adoring boyfriend, or at least to wake up with an adoring boyfriend who doesn't care that I don't have two normal legs.

At my new school, everyone assumes I'm an only child. I don't tell them that by the end of the year, I'll be a sister again, as Julie is coming home. She doesn't want to stay at school, so the nuns have found her a job in a chemist shop in Ormond. For the first time in years we will share a room. She is excited. I am nervous.

To compensate, we are given the best room, with a big bay window, Wavertree's only real asset. Mum insists that Dad builds a window seat, which he upholsters in thin nylon tomato-red velvet that wrinkles when you sit on it, and where Julie puts Annie May, her favourite doll, with her soft cloth body, big painted blue eyes and red felt bonnet. Dad builds us pine bunks, stained in Mum's favourite rosewood stain – offset with beading in her favourite colour – pillar-box red. We can't afford carpet so he covers the floor in mint-green lino.

"Wash the money off your hands," Mum tells Julie when she comes home from the chemist shop, wearing a white uniform zipped up the middle and copper-coloured eye shadow, her hair dyed a shade lighter and teased and curled around her face. Dad takes photos of us in the backyard with his new Polaroid camera, and we pose warily, side by side but apart.

Julie has two normal legs and lots of boyfriends. "Why does she bring all those boys home?" Mum says, when Julie brings them home, unannounced. I don't ask Julie where she gets them or what she does with them. During the day she is at the chemist shop, and on Friday nights she goes to Shindig, the local dance at the Mordialloc Life Saving Club. My papillomas are back and for much of that summer, I sit in the kitchen with my foot on a stool, watching Mum clean, cook and complain about Dad and the mess. Along with a boyfriend, I want a job as I have nothing to wear on "mufti day" at school. As soon as I recover, I get an after-school job at the local health food shop, where I blush and stammer as I pierce the bun on the thick metal spikes on the new hot dog machine, and struggle to fit the glistening red sausage into the hole.

It's me that Dad takes in the car now, to visit Gunter, his friend the staircase maker, and Darryl, his friend at the wood yard, who flirt with me, and Dad smiles when I blush and flirt back. It's me Dad takes on a dawn fishing trip at Black Rock with Aunty Mary's husband, Uncle Tony and my cousin Dom. We don't last long. I need the toilet and refuse to do it over the side of the boat, as Uncle Tony suggests. We come back with one small fish and one big dream.

"Dad and my project for the year is a yacht," I write in my diary the day before 1973 becomes 1974. Diaries for me usually begin on

January 1 and end on January 2, but that year I have a lot to write about.

The yacht is a Mirror, which comes in an easy-to-assemble kit and costs $300. Mum says it's a waste of money and Dad should wallpaper the hallway. I think it would be good for Mum to make friends with the other women at the yacht club, or maybe we should send her away for a holiday to visit her mythical cousin Dell in Sydney, whom none of us have ever met?

I abandon my attempts to play piano like Mum and ask to learn guitar, like Dad, who shows me how to hold it in the classical style, my foot on a metal pedal. Dad is making a guitar of his own – out of Mum's rosewood coffee table.

"Typical," says Mum, stepping over all the pieces of our washing machine, which Dad has taken apart to fix and failed to put back together, and in my mind I hear Nana Cafarella, with her throaty chuckle, describing how as a child, Dad would pull apart every toy car he got, and cry when he couldn't put them back together.

"Your blood's worth bottling," Mum says, as I pack our dirty washing in the grey plastic shopping jeep every week and lug it down to the local Laundromat. Dad's blood isn't worth "a pinch of shit" – not even when he buys a twin-tub washing machine, which staggers drunkenly all over the kitchen during the rinse cycle. Fed up, he pegs the clothes on the clothesline, rinsing them off with the hose. Mum rolls her eyes, but mine are wide with admiration.

"I did! I have! I will!" I snap, when Mum nags about homework or tells me to make my bed or sweep the floor. I feel bad. She's still sore from the hysterectomy, working part-time as a Hills Hoist representative at Myer in Frankston, selling rotary clothes hoists. But I'm distracted by my secret affair with my boss Rudy – at least that's my fantasy. Rudy looks like a Viking, with platinum hair and a beard like a copper scourer. When his wife Louise is out, Rudy writes his initials on my back with his finger. He wants to write them on my breast, but I won't let him. I am tantalised and guilty, flattered and terrified that Louise will find out and sack me, or that Rudy's attention will drift from my breasts to my legs, hidden in flared jeans and long Indian skirts.

I only confess this to my diary, and to my school friend Gail, who walks with Mini and me down to the beach after work, and where I sunbake with a towel hiding my big leg.

"Your leg is so white," Gail laughs, when I drop the towel and dash into the water.

Gail has a twin sister, Kirsten, who looks nothing like Gail, which makes us kindred spirits, as they don't get along either.

On New Year's Eve we are all invited to Aunty Iris's new house and orchard. The old house and orchard in Williamsons Road, have been sold to Westfield where they are building Doncaster Shopping Town.

"Julie and I will probably be dumped in the TV room. Aunty Iris always treats us as if we're about 12," I tell Dad.

"Ask her for a Monopoly set and a bottle of whisky," Dad says, and I laugh, feeling grown up.

The New Year feels old already as the patterns of previous years repeat. On Sunday mornings, Dad churns out mini life buoys of dough that drop into a sea of bubbling oil from our new donut machine. Mum has no appetite for donuts. "I'm sick of living in shit all my married life," she says, as she sweeps round the mess of buckets and paper in the hallway, which Dad and I are finally wallpapering.

I'm sick of it, too. Each day a tall boy called Stephen, with brown hair and a shy smile, comes into the shop where I work, asking for 20 cents worth of lollies – admiring the sweets I have to offer as I bend to pick out the mint leaves, raspberries and musk sticks he chooses. Eventually he asks me out, and I'm surprised when Mum says I can go, as long as I am home by nine.

"Aren't you hot?" he asks, as we walk to the beach together, my long blue skirt clinging to my legs. "No," I lie. "Long dresses are actually cooler."

The next day, he comes to pick me up on his pushbike, and insists I ride on the handlebars. The small galaxy of pimples on the sides of his cheeks glows crimson as he wobbles up the hill in Heslop Street, unaware that my big leg makes me a lot heavier than I look.

Weeks go by. I fend off kisses and questions, avoiding reasons to swim, to sunbake and to tell him I am born that way, until one day, after hauling me up the hill to his house, he takes me proprietorially by the hand and leads me upstairs to his small attic bedroom.

"You're beautiful," he says, and gently he lifts my top and gazes at my breasts, brown against my white bra.

"You're blind," I say pulling my top down.

"No, I'm not."

"Yes, you are."

"You're stupid," he says. "Come here," and he pulls me down on the bed and kisses me.

"I'm getting very fond of you, kid," he says.

"I'm not a kid," I say, and as if to test this theory he takes my hand and begins rubbing it gently against the mound growing in his brown cords.

Curious and fearful, I let him.

"Feel it," Stephen squeaks, small beads of perspiration forming on his upper lip as he pushes my hand down his pants, past prickly shrubbery, to where it touches a warm bar of flesh.

My hand closes over it. Stephen's eyes flutter and roll back in his head and his mouth opens slightly. I fear he'll pass out. It's first time I've felt an erect penis, but my mind isn't on the job. I'm too worried about what he'll see if he lifts my skirt.

He reaches up and fumbles with my bra strap.

"We'd better not."

Quickly, he retracts his hand.

"Sorry. Sorry," he says and we sit up and reassemble ourselves.

A week later I am waiting for the train to school, my legs exposed in my school dress, when a friend of Stephen's waves from the opposite platform. I wave back and slide my feet behind my school bag, my heart ricocheting in my chest. As soon as the train arrives,

I dash into the carriage and sink into the seat, sweating. That's it. I have to come clean.

"I've got something to tell you," I say as Stephen and I walk along the beach the following night.

He smiles. "Is it something nice?"

Oh no. Does he expect me to say I love him?

"No," I say hastily.

We walk in silence.

"Well, come on kid, out with it."

I can't. The relationship fizzles a few months later when Stephen gets a job in the city.

Mum and Dad's relationship is fizzling too. "So what do you want? A bloody medal?" Dad says, when night after night over dinner she regales us with tales of the terrible Mrs Tait, the floor manager at Myer, who is jealous of her sales record.

"And I hope it chokes you," Mum replies, slamming the meal down in front of him that she still feels obliged to cook.

Julie is packing to go to the Sunbury Pop Festival, which upsets Mum.

"Who will you go with? How will you get there? Where will you stay?" she asks.

"With friends," Julie says, answering all three questions at once.

While she is away, Nanny comes to stay, sleeping in Julie's top bunk.

"I never wanted you to marry him," Nanny says, distressed when Mum fights with Dad over Julie and all the disappointments of their life.

"The only reason you didn't want me to marry him was because he was foreign and not positioned enough," Mum says. "You were just as taken in by his flattery as everyone else."

On Sunday night, Julie comes home and throws herself and all her clothes into the bath.

"She's a real Cafarella. She's just like your father," Mum tells me, and when Dad comes home from work she hunts him down with her whittling and whining words as he flees from room to room.

At weekends Julie is mostly absent and everywhere I go in the house I stumble into walls of silence broken only on Sundays by Jack Little's Yankee drawl during World Championship Wrestling, which Dad watches in the lounge room.

"The hate is overpowering in this stadium tonight," Jack roars as Mario Milano and Killer Kowalski battle it out at Melbourne's Festival Hall.

"Tell your father lunch is ready," Mum says, blowing a wisp of hair from her bottom lip as she removes the roast from the oven.

Dad sits on the grubby yellow vinyl chair in his navy-blue shorts and white singlet, one muscular brown leg raised as he picks at the callous on his heel. The smell of orange peel and cigarette ash greets me and I'm just in time to see him raise his right buttock and emit a loud fart.

"There's a beauty, right to the point of the chin," Jack Little cries, as Killer Kowalski does the Jumping Knee Drop right on Mario's belly. Mario flips and pulls him into an angry embrace. Jack Little prises them apart and forces them to shake hands. He forces Killer's arm into a victory salute. The crowd goes wild.

Mum and I eat in silence in the kitchen, staring at the $20 note Dad has tucked under the plastic fluted sugar bowl for housekeeping.

At night, I confide in my diary.

Mum and Dad are fighting again. But I refuse to get involved. They'll have to work it out for themselves. If Mum decides to leave, I will go with her, because she needs me more.

But I am involved. All these years, she stayed "for the sake of you children", but she can't take it anymore, she just can't, she tells me late at night when Dad is at work.

"We're not children anymore," I say.

"How can I destroy the family?" she says.

"It's destroyed already."

"Where would I go? What would I do?" she asks, her eyes wild.

"You've got a job. I've only got one more year of school. We'll be all right."

Mum rings Dad's sister Tess for a second opinion. Dad rings Tess, too. Tess is going crazy. We are all going crazy until Tess lends Mum $60 to rent the flat in Spray Street for a trial separation. Julie doesn't come. "I asked her to come, but she chose HIM," Mum says.

And at the front of my diary, I cross out *1 Heslop St, Parkdale, 3194*, and replace it with *1A Spray St, Parkdale, 3194, as of 23/7/74*.

"Tell your father this," Mum says, when I go back to Heslop Street to collect the mail. "Tell your mother that," Dad says. Until one day Mum gives me a yellow envelope and says, "Tell your father I want a divorce."

I don't recall what my father says when I hand him that envelope. I assume, that like Mum and me, he's had enough of trying to make it work. I assume things will be as they always have been – Mum and I in one camp and Julie and Dad in the other. The only difference will be our separate houses, which we will traverse in the same way as other teenage children of divorced parents, rolling our eyes and sidestepping the nasty comments designed to tarnish the image of the absent parent.

It will be a relief to navigate these barbs occasionally instead of every day.

I will be free.

6

That summer, six months after Mum and I move out, Mum's sister Dottie invites us to stay for a week during the holidays to keep Nanny company. Dottie is the secretary at a prestigious private girls' school and when school is out, so is she. Pa died four years earlier, and Nanny lives in the flat they once shared in the backyard behind Dottie's big red brick house.

I am glad to be at Dottie's, free from the circular conversations with Mum about whether we've done the right thing by leaving Dad, and what will become of her now "after 20 years of hell, no money, ill-health and two sick children", now she's alone with no future and a teenager to support. And how she'd asked Julie to come with us, but Julie "chose HIM, which was not surprising since she was HIS all along".

I haven't seen Julie since. We live in different worlds. She is 18 and still at the chemist shop, except now she has a steady boyfriend called Peter who's a spray painter. I'm 17 and still at school and have two new jobs. Rudy has sold the health food shop and I'm working at Carpay's Milk Bar next door two days a week after school and at Mensland on Saturday mornings, where men rarely come, as it's women who mostly buy their clothes, and who come in for "a ball of wool" from the skein they've reserved.

While Mum is showering in Dottie's big house, I plan to get ahead on my HSC reading and improve my tan. I want to be a journalist, which means getting good marks for English. It's one of those typical Melbourne summer days that has lapsed into Spring and is cool and cloudy – hardly sunbaking weather. But it's school holidays and I'm free and determined to do summery things, so I lay the thin bathroom towel on the scabby patch of grass in front of Nanny's flat and sit down. Carefully, I arrange the second towel over my big leg and reach for the bottle of coconut suntan oil, oiling my belly, flat and brown against the green and white bikini. Anyone looking will find their eyes lingering for the right reasons.

My only job at Dottie's is to call Mum to come in from the bathroom in the big house when lunch is ready. You can't swing a cat in Nanny's bathroom in the flat, Mum says. She needs elbow room for the morning ritual of cursing her long wispy black hair, which has to be wrestled into the bun that sits on the back of her head like a curled cat.

The bathroom in the big house is musk-stick pink and on the pink vanity stretching the length of one wall are two Mason and Pearson real bristle hair brushes, engraved in swirly gold writing – SDB for Sophia Doris Barnett, which is Dottie, and PEB for Philip Edward Barnett, my cousin Pip, who is 24 and the only cousin still living at home. His sister, my cousin Pam is married, and their big brother Joel has moved to London. Their father, Da, has been dead 10 years.

Julie is seven and I am six, when we run up to the front door one Christmas, and are greeted by Dottie, white faced. Da has a headache and has gone to bed. Later we learn Da is in hospital with something called a tumour on the brain.

"Isn't it disgusting?" Mum says and she clicks her tongue as she tells everyone how Doris hired a nurse and went to work, and how between operations Da fixed the fence but put the nails in the wrong way and Doris made him pull them all out.

Then Da is no more and the washing-up roster near the sink in Union Road has four names instead of five. I miss Da and feel sorry for Dottie, who still laughs when she and Mum drink sherry together, tossing her head with her dark curls swept up in a French chignon, and still gives us birthday money every year. From then on Dad plays barman at the Union Road family parties.

I glance at the French doors to the darkened dining room where my handsome cousin Pip is playing endless games of patience. I have a crush on Pip. I know it's wrong. You aren't supposed to feel that way about a first cousin. But his dark poodle-like hair, dark eyes framed by Superman-style glasses, and slim hips hugged by his tight black leather motorcycle jacket, make me blush and stammer.

I roll on to my side to read more comfortably, carefully replacing the towel over my big leg. The morning sun refuses to come out and I am chilled. The cloying smell of warm meat wafts from the open door of the flat. It isn't long since breakfast but in Nanny's view a leg of lamb has to be incinerated before it's fit for human consumption.

Nanny is nearly 80 and has been for quite some time. "I'm nearly 80 and won't have much longer," she says whenever anyone upsets her. She suffers from rheumatism and bad "balance" and is so bandy Mum said she can't stop a pig in the street.

Bang! The wire door to the big house shudders. Mum is striding across the umbilical cord of grey pavers linking the big house to Nanny's flat. "Mum! Mum!" she cries. Her voice is shrill and startling, like the scream that escaped from the wounded rabbit Dad shot and failed to kill on our one and only camping trip.

"Mum!" she shrieks again. "Mum! Mum!"

Why is she calling Nanny? Have her thrombotic legs erupted like a bloody Vesuvius, as she always warned? No. Her long dark hair is loose and damp and her tomato-red nylon negligee billows behind her, exposing the rivers of chunky blue veins on her pale bare legs – intact.

She turns to me, her face knotted, "Jane! Get Pip! I want him to hear this," and the wire door of Nanny's flat smacks shut behind her. The towel falls to the ground as I scramble to my feet.

I have no memory of calling Pip or following my mother into the flat, but in my mind he is there, sitting on the dark wood Jacobean lounge chair with the tapestry cushions, beside the small round dining table neatly set for the lunch, as with her big bare feet, my mother paces the pink roses on the grey Axminster carpet.

"Where's Nanny?" she yells, her eyes darting around like a lion that's temporarily lost sight of its prey. "Mum!" she calls again.

Nanny appears, unsteady on her bandy arthritic legs, her face flushed from peering into the hot oven. Her blue-grey hair is as fine and fluffy as a dandelion and forms a small cloud above her forehead. Her dress is blue check to match her hair and her large breasts rest comfortably on the matching belt, secure in the knowledge that they have done their job and nothing more will be demanded of them. She wipes her hands on her apron and looks up, cloudy eyed. Nanny is nearly blind from cataracts. I once found her grinding a black shoelace to dust because she thought it was a spider.

"Lorraine!" she says in surprise, as if my mother is an unexpected visitor. "What's wrong?"

Mum waves a bulging white envelope in her face. "You knew!" she says, "You knew all along."

Nanny and I stare blankly at the envelope, which is fat like the envelopes Mum stuffs with the "Ticket-in-Tatts" lottery tickets she buys every week.

"I don't know what you're talking about," Nanny says.

"This!" Mum says, slamming the envelope on the dining room table, where it coughs up a flurry of paper torn in uneven strips. I recognise my father's neat slanting writing. Why has Dad written a letter, and why has someone torn it up?

Mum opens her left fist. Bits of torn letter fall to the table, and I realise she's pieced it together. Again, I wonder who tore up the letter and why. Mum recites slowly:

As I took the pins from your hair I realised I'd married the wrong sister.
"The wrong sister!"

The word "sister" struggles half-strangled from her throat.

Nanny falls shakily into a chair, her face crimson. There is panic in her cloudy blue eyes.

"Now, Lorraine …" she says.

Mum isn't listening.

"THAT'S why she wouldn't tell me where she was going," she yells. "She's with HIM! My own sister!"

Fluttering pieces of information gather in my brain like the pieces of the letter, as I try to work out what's happening. I know this scene. I've seen it in the book on Joan Sutherland, in my mother's bookshelf. A woman in a white nightgown streaked with blood, smiling strangely. The mad scene from Lucia di Lammermoor. Except my mother wears a blood-red nightgown and she's screaming, not smiling.

"You knew and you protected her," Mum yells, sitting heavily on the Jacobean couch, her head in her hands.

Nanny's face goes from white to pink to red. "I don't know what you're talking about."

"Don't play dumb with me. That's why she's not here," Mum says, her menopausal corned-beef complexion turning one shade darker. "On holiday my foot! She's with HIM. Don't tell me you didn't know."

The fluttering pieces of information begin to take form. HIM is my father. HER is my aunt, Dottie, Mum's sister. Dottie is with Dad. Dad is with Dottie. They are on holiday. Together.

I don't look at Pip. I only see my mother, circling. Nanny is defenceless in the face of my mother's rage, which fills the room like a noxious gas. I hold my breath, not wanting to inhale.

"I'm old. What was I to do?" Nanny pleads. She wipes her face on her apron, the face with skin so fine it can only tolerate the finest green Palmolive soap. She looks up, suddenly mean-eyed.

"Anyway, you didn't want him!"

And in my mind I heard Dottie saying, "At least you've got a man," when I am a child and Mum sits on Dottie's couch in Union Road, sipping Three Roses sherry and complaining about Dad.

Now Dottie has a man and it's my father.

Mum's fist lands in front of Nanny with a thud. Nanny jumps.

"It's not HIM I care about. It's HER, turning her back on me. And to think I was going to move closer to Doris when my marriage broke up."

She paces in small circles and I am embarrassed to see her breasts wobbling, loose and unsupported under the thin red nylon nighty, as she throws questions like poison darts.

"How long has this been going on? How long?"

"I don't know."

"Since before the separation?"

"I don't know. I don't know," Nanny says, shaking her head. Her voice wavers and I'm afraid she might faint or cry.

"Yes, you do," Mum screeches. "THAT'S why he agreed to the separation. SHE encouraged it. He's gone where he knew his bread would be buttered. And what have I got after 20 years of marriage? Nothing. No family, no money, nothing!" And she throws herself on the couch, gouging her forehead with her fingers.

"You've got family," Nanny cries.

"Who? Who?" Mum yells, gesturing to the empty dining chairs.

"Me!" I think, but I know I'm part of the problem, as I still have one year of school left before I can get a full-time job. My Aunt Tess may have lent us the money for a flat, but neither Tess nor anybody else has any money to help us further, or any room for us, even if they wanted to help. Besides, we are firmly aligned with Mum's side of the family.

"Where are they staying?" Mum demands, squinting at Nanny.

"I don't know," Nanny says.

"You must know. They wouldn't have gone without telling you. You're protecting her. You always protected her."

"Leave me alone. I'm nearly 80 and Dr McIntyre says I shouldn't get upset," Nanny says, and she hangs her head, defeated. "What was I to do? I'm old and have nowhere to go."

This is a truth Mum can't deny. Although Pa was a real estate agent, he and Nanny never owned their own home. Nanny owed the roof over her head to Doris and Da who'd built the flat for them when Pa retired.

But for Mum, there is another undeniable truth.

"She had everything, and now she's done this to me, who had nothing," she says stonily.

"You don't know what it's like to be a widow all these years," Nanny says, and once again, I am seven as Dad whispers "Don't tell Dottie I'm here," when I push the toilet door at Union Road open and find him hiding there at the party to farewell my cousin Joel when he goes to England to live.

Mum gives Nanny a cold stare. "So, she was lonely? Why didn't she get her own man? Why did she have to shit in my nest?"

"Who else knows?" she demands, her eyes narrowing. "Does Joel know? Does Pam know? If it's so right, why doesn't she tell THEM? Why doesn't she tell the world?"

Nanny doesn't know. Then she says no one knows, then everyone knows and she doesn't know why she is being attacked like this. She shakes her head, battered and bewildered: "Why can't you just forget him?"

Mum stares at her in disbelief and turns to me. "Jane! Get the phone book!"

I don't move. I've been so busy watching from the wings I forget my entrance.

"We're leaving. Get the phone book so we can call a taxi," she says.

Nanny looks up, startled. "Where are you going? Lorraine! Don't leave like this."

I stand, an automaton pressed into action, and fumble for the phone book. Like onion skins, the flimsy pages won't be separated. Mum snatches it, finds the number and calls the taxi – her voice calm and firm. I wonder how we will afford a taxi all the way from Balwyn to Parkdale.

Nanny stands shakily, grasping the edge of the table. "What about me? What will I tell them?"

"Ask Doris," Mum says.

I don't remember whether Pip leaves or stays to comfort Nanny in the flat. Everything else plays like a tape recorder in my head, but here the tape goes blank. I don't remember dressing or packing, just Mum and I standing at the door of the flat, fully clothed with our bags, and in a voice that is strangely normal, Mum tells Nanny, "Don't come out. It's too hot." And I realise the sun is out.

We walk in silence down the driveway and wait in front of the big house. My stomach growls. The smell of the roast we never ate hangs in the air, along with the smell of Mum's perfume – Tabu, which is the colour of sherry and comes in a red box with the picture of a man and woman, locked in a sensuous embrace.

I stare at the familiar scrunched cream satin blinds on the curved windows of the big house, the red brick steps where my sister Julie and I trod excitedly each Christmas, waiting to be swept into our uncle's arms; the low brick fence lined with camellias in winter and hydrangeas and roses in summer, tended by a gardener once a month, and where a pet tortoise once roamed.

He took the pins from her hair. I think of Dottie's black curly hair falling, and us falling with it.

From now on, it's The Ma and The Kid versus the Gigolo and the Monster, as Mum dubs Dad and Dottie.

From now on, this is the story that rewrites my life, the story of how I lose my whole family without anybody dying.

PART TWO

Searching

7

Saturday nights are the worst. The novelty of setting up the camp bed for me in the lounge room has long since worn off and the roof of our ground floor flat is so low it feels like an elephant is sitting on our heads. There's no school, no work and no friends or family. On Saturday nights, it's not The Ma and The Kid. It's just her.

"Here I am at the age of 47, with nothing and no one," she says as we stare at each other over the wobbly card table, opposite the white venetian blinds, closed to the world. Her words scare me. If she has nothing and no one, then neither do I.

"You've got me," I say.

In the wake of The Great Betrayal, as I now think of it, family and friends have abandoned us, or we have abandoned them. I'm not sure which. Either way my mother is too humiliated to face their judgement or pity.

"Nobody wants you when you've got no money and ill-health," she says.

"You don't have ill-health now."

She raises a sceptical eyebrow.

"There's nothing left," she says, gazing at the remnants of her former life.

"It'll be okay," I say, although I'm not sure how.

Until the house at Heslop Street is sold we have no money, other than from my afterschool jobs in Parkdale and her part-time earnings at Myer, where she is working in the gift department. Forced to leave school at 16, when her father was called up by Manpower during the War to work in a munitions factory in the city, she has no real skills, other than "selling ice to Eskimos", which is how she describes her success in sales.

There's no food in the house either.

"Let's go out for dinner," I say. I have $20 saved. My treat.

"On our own?"

"Why not?"

"Where will we go?"

"To the city"

"At this hour?"

"Everything's open late in the city."

By the time we get to Flinders Street, everything is shutting. The few people around are heading home, not out. Those who linger are mostly sharpies – gangs of youths with shaved heads and mullets – and "derros" as Mum calls the homeless men sleeping in the phone booths.

"It's too late," she says, as we wander down Bourke Street.

"There's a place," I say, pointing to a tiny café in a small arcade lit by a cold fluorescent light, where a weary waiter is putting chairs upside down on the tables.

"Are you open?" I ask. They aren't. "Do you know of any other place that's open?" They don't. The waiter sighs and turns two chairs right side up. They make us scrambled eggs in a silver skillet, but not with dry curds the way Mum makes it.

"Isn't this terrible?" she says poking the glistening glob of congealed yellow vomit.

"At least you're not cooking," I say poking mine. I hate runny eggs.

She looks up at the blinking Tivoli sign in the arcade, a nod to its past life as the famous Tivoli Theatre, specialising in variety acts and vaudeville.

"I won the Tivoli Competition. I did," she says. The "I did" is a form of rhetorical punctuation she favours whenever she is dazzled by her own audacity, like the time she organised a concert for the war effort when she was only 11. "I hired the hall, organised all the acts. Everything. I did!"

"I know."

I know this story and the story of how she'd won the Tivoli's "search for a star".

"I entered the Tivoli Competition for a joke. They wanted me to tour, but I wasn't interested. I was more interested in opera," she says, as we leave and the waiter puts our chairs back on the table. I know this too. She was destined for better things. Like Covent Garden.

"Thorold Waters, *The Sun* newspaper music critic, came in a taxi to persuade Nanny and Pa to let me go to Covent Garden with him. But they were against it," she tells me again.

Their war-hero son Joel was dead. Doris was married. Lorraine was all they had left.

"You should have gone," I say as we walk back to Flinders Street station.

She shakes her head. "You didn't go against your parents in those days."

"There's a price for everything," she says, meaning the hefty price she has paid for her rebellion.

* * *

The blue train on the way home is almost empty. We sit facing each other, staring at our flickering reflections in the darkened windows as the suburbs rush by. I watch as it begins, her new habit of chewing the left side of her lip. As if to draw attention to her internal hurt, she has created an external wound she is compelled to pick and poke at, and which I regard as an affectation and an embarrassing plea for attention.

"Stop it," I say.

"What?"

"Chewing your lip."

"Was I chewing my lip?"

A minute later she begins again.

"Stop it."

"All right, I won't do it," she says, like a repentant child. But, of course, she does, more frantic than before, watching me, challenging me to say something. I feign disinterest as her lip turns from pink to red, until we alight at Parkdale Station and her face is absorbed by the darkness as we walk home.

Inside the flat, Mum retreats to the bathroom as I set up my bed in the lounge room.

The phone rings. Mum darts back into the lounge room, her black hair loose and fanned around her shoulders. She shoots me a look and answers with a cautious "Hello?"

A faint high-pitched voice squeaks away in compressed fury.

Mum slams down the phone and sinks into the rocking chair.

"She's been drinking," she says in disgust. SHE is Doris – The Monster – from whom random late-night calls are another part of our Saturday night routine.

"Why is she doing this? She got what she wanted. Why can't she leave me alone?" Mum says, sucking on her cigarette like a dying person sucking oxygen.

"She's nuts," I say.

It's hard to imagine Doris saying anything to my mother other than "G'day Nipper," a habit from their childhood. She never calls her Lorraine. The nickname feels like a reminder of Mum's status as the youngest child. Born Lorraine Jean Hill in 1928 on the cusp of the Great Depression, her arrival demoted the six-year-old Doris to middle child and promoted their eight-year-old brother Joel to hero.

"I loved my brother. He taught me things," Mum says as our conversation shifts from Doris, The Monster, to Joel, the God. A Navigator with the 10th Sunderland Squad in the Australian Airforce, Joel was shot down in the Bay of Biscay in 1943 when Mum was 15. Reduced to a sepia photo on Nanny's mantlepiece in

Florence Street, he is both young and old, wearing the war service dress uniform and peaked cap reserved for air crews.

Two years later, another photo appears – of Doris in a white satin wedding dress, surrounded by a coronet of smiling bridesmaids. A year later their dead brother is resurrected when Doris names her first son after him. Two more children follow – my cousins Pip and Pam. People begin to talk: why isn't there a photo of Lorraine in a white satin dress on the mantelpiece? She is, after all, 24.

Lorraine is too busy learning to be an opera singer at the newly formed National Theatre Opera School founded by opera singer Gertrude Johnson, who returns from an illustrious career in London appalled by the lack of opportunities for young singers. Mum's cousin Dell – Aunty Iris's sister – is at the adjoining National Theatre Drama School. Between shows, they escape to Sydney, staying in boarding houses and picking up office work, the distant sound of church bells reminding them of the lives they were meant to lead. Until Nanny insists that Mum returns to Melbourne.

"Dance with me, go out with me, marry me," a handsome Jewish man pleads, the one time Mum deigns to go to a dance in St Kilda where the other girls go husband hunting, and he takes her to see a house he is building.

"I should have married the Jew," Mum says, reaching for the sherry bottle.

"What was his name?" I ask again, wondering who I might be if she had. She shakes her head. She can never remember. He wasn't a person but a symbol of the life she might have had.

"I wasn't ready," she says, draining her glass.

Not until June 1955, when she marries my father, Francesco Ambrosia Maria Bartolomeo Cafarella. She's 27. He's 22. She's Australian. He's Italian. She's Anglican. He's Catholic. It's perfect.

They marry in the vestry of St Patrick's Catholic Church in Mentone. A church wedding is not allowed.

There are only two photos of the wedding. Neither makes it to Nanny's mantelpiece at No. 42 Florence Street. In the first, Mum wears a white fascinator on her cropped hair and a pale suit, which she tells me was duck-egg blue. The suit has three-quarter sleeves, accentuating her long arms.

My father wears a black suit and a boyish grin. They stand behind a modest cake, flanked by Nanny Hill and Nana Cafarella, wearing hats and fox furs, raising a champagne toast – the only photo I ever see of my two grandmothers together. In the second photo, someone holds an umbrella as Mum slides into a waiting car with her new husband.

It's on her honeymoon that she realises her mistake. "I heard them page Mrs Cafarella, and I didn't answer," she tells me again.

"So why did you marry him?" I ask for the millionth time. And for the millionth time, she says, "I thought he had potential," as if she's talking about a prospective employee.

"I thought I'd get out of it after a while," she says – as if getting out of it was as easy as stepping out of a dress. Other times she claims it was an act of rebellion for Nanny and Pa's refusal to let her go to Covent Garden.

The stories of the lost dream and the ill-fated marriage are added to the stories of the severed fingers and the cleaving. There are other stories I can't know, as my mother reminds me as we sit together in our small flat with our new smaller life.

"You don't know the half of it," she says, regarding me sadly.

I don't. All I know is that I am 17 and she is 47 and we are alone with nothing and no one. As night turns to morning, once more, I put my hand in hers and I understand.

8

Twenty Saturday nights later, I go to church. Not to pray, but to worship Michael Lawry, the Adonis of the Cheltenham Church of Christ Youth Club with my friend Gail, who has invited me.

Except Gail doesn't turn up. I don't know anyone else. It's one year since Mum and I have split from Dad and Julie. We're still living in Spray Street, Parkdale, and Mum is home reading her new Bible, Linda Goodman's Sun Signs, confident that I'm in wholesome company. I think about going home, but the charismatic minister herds all those who have turned up into a convoy of cars headed for his holiday house in Dromana for a wholesome church barbecue. It's a balmy summer night. I don't know where Dromana is, or the name of the boy driving the car or the names of any of the other three young people in the back seat with me as we hurtle down Balcombe Road.

We ram into each other as the car swerves into the driveway of a two-storey brown clinker brick house. The young driver hangs his head out the window and addresses a smiling boy sitting astride a motor bike, his helmet tucked under his arm.

"Hey, Dale. Wanna come to a barbie in Dromana?"

"Okay," the boy says, and he hangs his helmet on the handlebars of the bike and squeezes into the backseat next to me.

I forget about Gail and Michael Lawry, as Dale's leg presses firm and warm against my good leg.

I soon learn that Dromana is on the coast, about an hour from Mentone along the Nepean Highway, and that being in the backseat of a strange car with Dale is kismet, verified when Dale quips that we are *Strangers in Paradise*, like the song, which I know comes from the movie *Kismet*. It's fate, sealed by the fact that Dale's house, where he parked his motorbike, is right opposite Aunty Mary's, although I don't admit that, not after Dale jokes about the crazy Italian family across the road. I haven't seen Aunty Mary since before Mum and Dad separated, so technically we're no longer related.

I haven't seen or heard from Dad either. Nor do I expect to. Any contact would be a further betrayal of my mother. Just as he and Mum are divorcing, so are we. I don't care. That's a past life. The present is a broad shoulder leaning against mine, dark eyes gazing into mine, and the unfamiliar scent of aftershave and bristling masculinity.

Dale is 20 and a junior real estate agent. He is surprised that I'm 17 and still at school. "You look older," he says, which I regard as a compliment. While the church minister doles out sausages and bread in Dromana, Dale and I circle each other around the pool table. I tell him I want to be a journalist and he asks me if I read Phillip Adams.

"Phillip who?" The only newspaper that ever enters our house is *The Listener In*, bought for the television guide and for wrapping the vegetable peelings. Dale offers to give me some of Phillip's articles. By the end of the night Dale has my phone number and I have an invitation to a party the following Saturday.

As soon as I say yes, I wish I'd said no. Like Cinderella, I have nothing to wear. More particularly I have no suitable shoes. Apart from black lace-up school shoes, the only shoes I own are a pair of mismatched thongs and the blue canvas men's shoes I wear with jeans and flares at weekends. My right foot is too big to fit anything else.

As the date with Dale looms, the need for a magical shoe solution grows urgent.

"I found a place in Windsor that has extra wide fittings," Mum says one night, eyeing me over the white cat's-eyes' glasses she's painting with hot pink nail polish. Shoe shopping was an annual ordeal when I was a child – to be avoided. But I don't want to say no to Dale.

"What's your widest fitting?" Mum asks the young shop assistant, as we examine a beige Mary Jane shoe on the stand at the wide-shoe shop in Windsor the following Saturday.

"Triple E," the girl says.

"Do you have it in a 10?" Mum asks

The girl nods, her eyes widening to a quadruple E as I place my big foot in its white sock on the metal measuring plate.

"We'll need two different pairs," Mum says, in a voice that warns ask at your peril, and the girl scuttles off to find my size.

The pungent smell of new leather wafts up at me when she returns and lifts a shoe the size of a small canoe from its bed of tissue paper, stretching the middle with her hand until it yawns and gapes before placing it before me. The mouth of the shoe gags as I lower my foot into it, and once again I am seven years old at the local ballet class, feeling the outrage of a dozen astonished eyes as I try to cram my big foot into a ballet shoe the size of a slivered almond.

"We'll try the 11, shall we?" the girl says, and she disappears again. The size 11 is a small dinghy, but still too narrow. Tomorrow night is my first date with Dale and I'll be wearing men's runners under my dress.

"I'm so sorry," she says. "You could try a surgical boot maker."

Surgical bootmakers make sturdy lace-up boots for people with funny feet and callipers, not shoes, and certainly nothing for a party. Mum asks where such a surgical bootmaker might be found. "Try the city," the girl says.

After an hour of traipsing around the city, we give up.

"We can have lunch at Cole's, if you like?" Mum says.

My foot is tight and aching from all the walking. I'm glad to sit down at the busy Cole's cafeteria while she queues for a sandwich and a pot of tea for her and a pie and lemonade for me. The pie is hot and burns my tongue and as I reach for the lemonade, the tears I don't want for the shoes I can't find pour down my cheeks.

"I'm a freak," I splutter.

Mum puts down her teacup and regards me with alarm. She waves grandly towards the crowds of people shuffling carefully past with their abundant clattering trays.

"There's a freak," she cries pointing to a woman juggling a tray of milk shakes.

"Look, there's a freak," she says, pointing to a man hunched over a sandwich. "There's a freak," she announces to one surprised shopper after another, until I burn with embarrassment. I want to shout at her to stop, but I'm too ashamed. She's trying to help, but she can't. No one can. I'd seen my future when I was nine, when I stumbled across a photo in our Pears' Encyclopaedia – of a woman with a leg so big the skin on her thigh fell in great plum-coloured folds like a curtain. "Elephantiasis", the caption read. I slammed it shut, my scalp prickling with horror. From then on, I feared that, like Alice in Wonderland who drinks from the bottle labelled "Drink Me" and grows so big she can't fit in the White Rabbit's house, no shoe and no house will ever be big enough to accommodate my foot.

I pick up the remaining pie with trembling hands.

Mum pours herself another cup of tea, as all the freaks she's identified walk on, oblivious.

"Your father and I were talking before we left, about getting a medical opinion."

A medical opinion? I stare stupidly, the pie suspended.

"Just to see if anything can be done. You never know these days. But you have to finish school first."

The notion that my parents ever talked about anything other than their failing marriage amazes me. Yet here she is, calmly telling me there's a specialist who may be able to help.

Fresh tears threaten. I can barely finish my pie. I know there's only a one-in-a million chance that anything can be done, but one in a million is better than nothing.

I don't tell anyone, not even Gail. It seems too improbable. But later that night, as I lie in bed, I think about what it will be like not to be me: to be free to choose any shoe.

Two days later Mum comes home from work with more good news. She's seen some shoes called Homyped in a chemist shop. They may be suitable. I barely look up from my homework. Homyped sounds suspiciously like surgical boots. She hands me a pamphlet. The shoes are white with thick platform soles and two thick straps across the top, fastened with adjustable silver buckles. The straps can be extended for my big foot, she says.

Platform shoes are in. I smile.

That's one problem solved. I have no idea how to solve the other one.

I'd already had two boyfriends when we were living in Heslop Street. I know that, eventually, they not only want to see your legs but everything above and below, just like Stephen my first boyfriend when I was 16 – and Paul.

Paul was a fellow team member at the local badminton club where I played weekly, and was as perfect as a store manikin, with wavy black hair, dark eyes and olive skin. Badminton and table tennis were the only sports I was good at, although they made my foot swell and ache. I ignored it, focusing on the looks I got when I tossed my long hair back as I bent to flip the shuttlecock onto my racquet. I ignored the coach's pleas to wear a short white dress and white sandshoes too, pointing out that the soles of my blue canvas shoes were white and I would get a dress soon.

One night the manikin spoke to me. "Do you want to go to the drive-in some time?"

"Yes," I said, elated.

"Come home straight after," Mum said.

I wore my jeans with the buttons on the sides, impossible to remove in a car. As soon as the movie started, Paul reached over and began to kiss me. Stephen's kisses were a mutual exchange of drool, flavoured with hamburger, but Paul's kisses were soft, warm and dry. He broke off and sunk low into his seat, unzipping his pants. Out popped his penis, as slim and brown as its owner. Something was expected. But what?

"Kiss it."

Kiss it? I hesitated, awaiting clearer instructions.

"Kiss it," he repeated, and slipping his hand behind my neck he pushed my head towards where a small tear was forming in the tiny slit at the top. I resisted. A tissue was clearly required.

"It's all right. I've got some wet checks in the glove box," he said.

Cheques were things that bounced. I'd never heard of wet checks. They sounded like Wettex, the yellow sponges Mum used in the kitchen. I shook my head. Better safe than sorry. Paul frowned and prised his penis back into his jeans, where it formed a sideways bulge. My face burned as we watched the rest of the film in silence. I'd been spared.

The following week, our badminton team was competing at our first inter-club tournament in Albert Park. A white dress was compulsory.

"How short do you want it?" Gail's mother asked as she pinned the hem of the dress with the sweetheart neckline she had offered to make.

"Not too short," I said, and in my mind I screamed, "Long. Hide me."

On the night of the tournament, I stood in front of the bay window in my bedroom in Heslop Street in the evening light, staring at my reflection in the mirror, wearing the white dress that revealed my secret. A low wolf whistle pierced the air. It was Dad, outside in the front yard from where my room was illuminated. It didn't help. He could only see me from the waist up.

At the stadium I sat on the benches that hugged the walls. Everyone else was on the court warming up. Sick with dread, I pulled off my jeans, picked up my racquet and walked to the front of the court. Across the net, my opponents' eyes expanded like balloons as they travelled from my thigh to my right foot in its size 11 men's blue canvas shoe, the white lace stretched so far there was no lace left to form a bow.

I took a deep breath. I knew what to do. I stuck out my chin and gave them the same look I'd seen Mum give the shop assistants over the years when we were shoe shopping – ask at your peril, stare at your peril – the look that had shielded us both then and which shielded me now. The whistle blew. The shuttlecock hurtled towards me. I jumped up. Whack! It flew over the net. Cheers.

After the tournament, I went quietly back to the safety of my jeans.

Six months have passed since that night. The Paul problem has now been replaced with the Dale problem.

9

"Nervous?" Dale says, as we stand at the front door of a modest weatherboard house in Heathmont. We are about to take our relationship to the next level. I am about to meet his sister.

"Yes," I say, and he gives me an encouraging kiss.

I take a sly peep at my feet. That afternoon, with a can of spray-on shoe dye, I transformed the white Homypeds to match my new brown flared cords. An hour before Dale is due to pick me up, the paint is still sticky. I wear them anyway, hoping they'll dry as the night progresses.

Dale's sister Laura is slim and blonde and the proud owner of a new husband and a new house. We sit on the floor as she spreads the photos of her wedding and honeymoon over the new beige carpet. Sitting on the floor is difficult, as my right leg doesn't bend easily. I tuck my legs behind me, leaning on one hand, feigning interest in the wedding dress.

As we rise to go to dinner, Laura pauses and leaves the room, returning with a cloth and a small bottle. She points to a brown smudge on the carpet. "Sorry, but can you all please check your shoes? I think someone might have trod in something."

I blush and try to check the soles of my Homypeds without anyone seeing my feet. All clear. Laura frowns, opens the bottle, turns it upside down on the cloth and, dropping to her knees, begins working the liquid into the stain. My heart pounds as the smudge spreads.

"It's not coming out," she says, puzzled.

I don't enlighten her. It's a temporary problem. In six short months, at the end of the school year, I'll have a new leg and new shoes.

Earlier that month, Bernard McCarthy O'Brien, a world-famous micro surgeon with steely grey hair, steely eyes and a steel-grey suit, had examined my leg in his rooms at East Hill House, next to St Vincent's Private Hospital, his finely boned hands gently pressing here and there, creating temporary indentations, until, satisfied, he spoke his diagnosis into a small black tape recorder: "Patient Jane Cafarella. Seventeenth of the ninth fifty-seven, presents with chronic lymphoedema of the right leg – Milroy's Disease."

Milroy's disease? Lymphoedema? I turned the strange words over in my mind. It was the first time my problem had a name – and it was as ugly as my leg.

"I can help you, but your leg will never be normal," Mr O'Brien said, fixing me with his steely gaze. "Do you understand? There will be scars."

My heart danced. Scars were normal. Scars could be explained. Lots of people had scars. Bring on the scars!

Mum and I listened as Mr O'Brien explained his plan to reconnect the lymph vessels in my groin with the blood vessels, in the hope that they would find new drainage paths. If that failed, he would do a series of operations to cut away the fibrotic lymphatic material, reducing the size of my leg. "There will be scars," he repeated.

There will also be bills, which our health insurance won't pay as my condition is "pre-existing". But Mr O'Brien pleads my case and schedules the operation for the week after my HSC exams.

The money from the sale of Heslop Street has finally arrived and we have moved to a two-bedroom flat in Davies Street, Mentone, a short walk from school.

"Your mother could make a home out of a tin shed," Nanny says, when she surveys the eclectic range of second-hand furniture from the local op shop.

The new flat means Mum needs a fulltime job to pay the extra rent and health insurance. The money from the sale of Heslop Street was "a pittance" and she has no money left to speak of.

"No one will employ a woman my age," she says as she runs her finger over the job ads in the local paper.

Nanny says she should get a man not a job.

"Oh, Mum! No man would want me," Mum says – and the pain in her eyes gives me a pain in my heart.

"And what would they say about my marriage?" she pleads. "They'd run a mile when they found out what that Gigolo and that Monster did to me. It was terrible, wasn't it? Wasn't it terrible?"

As she leaves, Nanny hands us each an envelope with 20 dollars saved from her pension. "Oh Mum, you shouldn't," Mum says,

"Well, you need it more than I do," Nanny says, and she heads jerkily down the stairs on her bandy legs to the waiting taxi, with her usual farewell of "Hoo roo!"

"I'm a failure," Mum tells me after Nanny leaves, and she reaches for *Linda Goodman's Love Signs*, which has replaced *Linda Goodman's Sun Signs*, and which explains everything.

"It wasn't your fault," I say. "Age is no barrier if you're good at your job. You're the best salesperson Myer's got."

She regards me cynically, a signal for me to launch a familiar script: she isn't a failure; she's the biggest success I've ever known. She isn't too old. She doesn't look old at all. She looks great. And why does she need a man at all?

To further convince her, the next month, when she turns 48, I celebrate by writing her a five-page letter thanking her for all she's done for Julie and me and championing her escape from her marriage.

The trouble was even if you stayed, you could not be sure that the self-sacrifice would be in vain. You tried, but how can you build a

relationship with someone if that someone is destroying himself and everyone around him? Impossible, and Mum, no one can ever achieve the impossible.

And I reassure her that Dad and Doris's betrayal is not her fault.

The important thing is that she's on the road to recovery from her broken marriage and life.

"Your blood's worth bottling," she says, when she reads it.

In the following weeks, she begins to comment that she'd always promised herself a facelift before she turned 50, until it begins to feel like a right she's been waiting to claim.

She complains of painful polyps in her nose and disappears one day for a "minor procedure", requiring her to wear heavier make-up and a headscarf covering her ears for the next two weeks. Along with the polyps, the bone in her nose is removed, which is shortened and squished at the tip. New false teeth appear, iridescent white and doll-like, giving her a horsey look, until they settle into her mouth. Evenings are spent at the suntan salon across the road, until bit-by-bit all her freckles from childhood join up, giving her the same hue as her favourite wood stain – rosewood. She begins to pick at her food and her round hips became angular. And as if released from hiding, a dimple appears on her right cheek.

While I scour shops for clothes that are concealing, she scours them for clothes that are revealing.

I try not to look shocked as she prances from bedroom to bathroom in nothing but her lacy black bra and panties, no longer my mother but a very old teenager. I try not to look shocked when she finds a boyfriend, a widower called Jim, with three teenage sons, whom she meets at Parents Without Partners, which I regard as a social club for desperate divorcees.

While my mother's body is shrinking mine is busting out. "There you are, all tits and teeth," she says when I show her my class photo, my breasts emphasised by my tight polo jumper. Recognising we are no longer girls, the school allows Year 12 students to wear casual clothes.

We are both at school now. I'm studying for my Higher School Certificate. Five subjects are recommended, but I drop History because it clashes with English Literature, my favourite subject. My free periods are spent watching *Ivan's Midday Movie* with Gail while discussing our other favourite subject – boys.

Mum is an unwilling student at Stott's Business College in the city, where with the help of Gough Whitlam's National Employment and Training Scheme, she hopes to get a full-time office job.

"I hate that bloody school in there," she says, as she cooks dinner, banging down the pots for emphasis. "It's the most dehumanising horrible atmosphere I've ever been in. It concentrates on petty things. It makes me feel like a complete idiot. I wish I'd never started that bloody course."

I wish she hadn't either. It's 1975, The Year of the Woman, but to Mum, all women are untrustworthy competitors.

"All those women. Women everywhere. And they fight like cats." She glares at me. "And then I come home to women. God Almighty! (Bang). Don't you ever tell me that you can cope with the working world." (Slam). You haven't been anywhere or done anything yet. It's so protected in there. (Bang). Let's see how you fare when you get a job and have to earn your own living. (Slam)."

A cold fear washes over me. Will I get a job? What if I fail HSC, destroying my chances to be a journalist? I'm doing well at English and English Literature, which I hope will compensate for French, which I only picked up in Form Three. At my previous school, we studied Indonesian, but now "Baik tarima kasih", is being replaced with "Merci beaucoup", and "l'amour" with Dale.

"I hope you're being careful," Mum says, as we preen together in front of the bathroom mirror on Friday nights before our respective dates. I look forward to this weekly ritual: the sticky sweet smell of perfume, hair spray and freshly ironed clothes, and the banter between rooms as we discuss what we're wearing and where we are going.

Of course, I lie about where Dale and I are going. I have to. I seldom know myself. Once it's to a place called Tiger's Eye, where we lie on brightly coloured cushions on the floor in a drowsy haze of smoke as Dale traces a slow line from my lips to my breast. Other times it's to the pub with friends.

"If anyone asks how old you are, tell them you're 18," Dale says, as two female police officers circle the Ladies' Lounge at the Beaumaris Hotel, where he's also teaching me how to drink tequilas. I nod, even though I won't be 18 for another six months. Sometimes, we go to see his friends Leslie and Nick, who live in a rented house in Mentone with a black dog called Gandalf, and who seem to be permanently curled up together on an old couch, smoking.

"Those cigarettes really stink," I say the first time I visit, waving my hand across my face and screwing up my nose as Leslie passes around a home-made cigarette, like the "rollies" Dad made from a blue wallet of Drum tobacco when I was a child. I don't smoke and have never been tempted. These smelly roll-your-owns, where you have to suck hard, seem hardly worth the effort.

Dale smiles and signals for me to meet him in the backyard.

"Those cigarettes are dope – or marijuana," he says. I'm not to worry. It's not dangerous. But I'm not to tell anyone either, and as if to seal the deal, he kisses me. I kiss him back, to show I understand. Other nights they pass around a bamboo cylinder full of water with a little bamboo pipe sticking out the side.

"Wanna have a go?" Nick asks.

"No," I say.

The acrid smoke they exhale is already creeping down my throat, but the look on Dale's face tells me this is a rite of passage I can't refuse.

"Not like that," he says, when I gasp and choke, and he shows me how to inhale slowly. On Saturday nights, we join Leslie and Nick on the couch, watching their sleepy satisfied smiles while they watch ours. It doesn't feel wrong. I feel safe with Dale, who not only has a job as a real estate agent but also plays guitar, though I never hear him play. When I finally turn 18 in September, he brings his new electric guitar to show me and Mum. I ignore Mum, who looks pointedly from the big new electric guitar to his birthday gift for me – a tiny bottle of Avon perfume, with the magic name of "In Love."

Nor does it feel wrong when later, when we are alone, Dale hands me a clear plastic bag full of marijuana seeds. He doesn't say what to do with them, so I shove them in the back of my underwear drawer in the tallboy in my bedroom.

On Saturdays, after we smoke with Leslie and Nick, we eat, and after we eat Dale and I drive down to Rickett's Point along Black Rock beach, where we make out in his blue Volkswagen Beetle, parked under the ti-tree bushes.

"What do you want to listen to?" he asks, setting the mood. I don't know. Apart from the Cat Stevens album of *Tea for the Tillerman* and Elton John's *Goodbye Yellow Brick* Road, bought on Stephen's recommendation, the world of pop music has passed me by.

"And you like that sort of music?" Mum asks, whenever I attempt to change the radio dial from ABC Classics.

Now I have a friend in James Taylor, Carol King and Pink Floyd and Dale, who doesn't seem to notice my legs – so far.

One night he announces we are going on a midnight picnic. The waves slap the shore and a cliché full moon illuminates the picnic rug he lays on a grassy patch near the Rickett's Point Tea House at Black Rock beach. Dale produces a bottle of wine and some cheese and crackers, and slowly peels off my top along with the cheese wrappers, before unwrapping the final delicacy, pulled from his pants, which he holds for me to admire.

I stare.

"Don't be afraid of it," he says.

Before I have a chance to explain exactly what I'm afraid of, there's a rustle in the ti-tree bush behind us.

"Shit! Someone's watching!" Dale says and he snatches the corners of the rug and we race back to the car.

Saved again.

A few weeks later he invites both Mum and me out for dinner, which seems sophisticated and gentlemanly and impresses us both. Over the white tablecloth in a little Italian restaurant in Edithvale, he talks of his plans to visit a commune in Nimbin with his friend Andrew, and I talk about my plans to write to all the big daily newspapers to ask about journalism cadetships.

"You should go to Learning Exchange," Dale says, and he explains it's a community newspaper that relies on volunteers – good experience for an aspiring journalist. Afterwards, Dale drops Mum home to our flat in Davies Street and we go to a party. Supposedly.

We park at Rickett's Point, not far from the teahouse. Dale pushes the front seats as far forward as they'll go. As the sun sinks and the light becomes shadowy, we climb into the back seat and remove each other's clothes. If he notices my leg, he doesn't say anything. He crouches smiling, naked before me, and for the first time I want it to be my first time. Dale is careful. Very careful. He doesn't wear a "raincoat". He wears a marquee in the form of two condoms.

We go "all the way" as *Shine on You Crazy Diamond* plays over and over. Weekend after weekend.

10

Shortly after our night of passion in the blue Volkswagen Beetle, Dale and I are standing alone on a balcony at a party, drinks in hand, when he leans into my neck and whispers the three little words I long to hear: "I love you."

"What did you say?" I ask.

I don't believe him. How can he love such imperfection?

Flushed and confused, he repeats it, then sips his beer and looks down at his shoes. The moment is lost, but I am determined to regain it during our holiday in the Victorian High Country in Dale's new Triumph sports car, which replaced the blue VW Beetle where I was de-flowered.

While Gail and my fellow Year 12 students are hunkering down in "Swot Vac" preparing for the October Tests before the final exams in November, I'll be swotting up on sex. I arrive early on Friday night, ready for our adventure, and am surprised to see Dale packing his gear into a plain, square, decidedly inelegant, unromantic old Volkswagen stationwagon.

"Where's the Triumph?"

"Sold," Dale says. "This is better for camping."

I'm disappointed. I imagined myself like Princess Grace, the tail of an elegant headscarf rippling gently behind me as the hoodless Triumph wound its way through picturesque scenery.

It hasn't taken much to convince Mum that I'm doing well in all my regular tests at school and will double my efforts after the holiday with Dale.

She's going on holiday with her boyfriend, Jim, to see if he's husband material. The best husbands are "comfortable" and "biddable". Jim qualifies on the first count, but I'm not sure he qualifies on the second. He always decides their social schedule and whenever he comes to pick up Mum he walks into our furniture and doesn't seem to notice how she stiffens at his clumsy fawning.

In my bag, I have the $50 Mum scraped together for food and expenses for my trip, but not the other thing that Dale asked me to bring.

"Did you get the pill?" he says, turning to me as we zigzag down the Omeo Highway, in the old station wagon, accompanied by the feverish strains of Stephane Grappelli.

"I forgot."

A shadow passes over Dale's face, while a blush rises in mine. I'm 18 and officially an adult, but I'm too scared to go to the doctor for a prescription for fear Mum will find out. Asking her for help never occurs to me, or that she must know exactly what we're doing. I stare ahead at the spiralling road, hoping Dale has brought condoms.

A week later, on the last leg of our trip, my money runs out. "Why didn't you bring more?" asks Dale, as he breaks the Cherry Ripe he bought for himself in half, and we eat in silence.

Mum greets me with a stern look when I return.

"You have marijuana in your drawer," she says, and from behind her back she produces the forgotten plastic bag of seeds, found when she put my clean underwear away.

"I thought you had more sense," she says, spitting the words at me.

How did she even know what they were?

She gives me a withering look. "I didn't come down in the last shower."

I plead for a return to grace, promising to see less of Dale, less of Gail and less of Ivan and his midday movie. That's easy. Gail has abandoned Ivan for last-minute study and Dale is slowly abandoning me. Since the holiday, our visits to Rickett's Point have become perfunctory. We "do it", and he drives me home in silence. Worse still, he drives me straight home and I drag myself from the car leaden with humiliation and rejection. I'm heartbroken but not surprised when he breaks it off, with a parting bottle of Avon *Unforgettable* perfume and a card: "Go on to better things, darling."

Worser things are more likely. I haven't done well in the October tests, held the week after my return from Omeo, and there are just three weeks before the final exams. I pin my hopes on doing well in the interviews for cadetships at *The Herald and Weekly Times*, which focus on current affairs. Gough Whitlam has just been sacked and the nation is in shock. I've studied it, written about it and discussed it endlessly in school. I'm ready.

Bill Hoey, the cadet counsellor who interviews me at *The Herald*, surveys me coolly, making a small cage with his fat white hands. "Cafarella – that's Italian, isn't it?"

I nod.

"What's the situation in Italy?"

Italy? Italy? I can hardly find it on a map.

I don't fare much better at *The Age*. Successful candidates will be notified soon, they say. But I already know the answer. My only hope is to do well enough in the final exams to get the 300 points for entry into the journalism degree at RMIT. I drag a kitchen chair onto the balcony outside the flat and balancing my typewriter on my knee, I type out all my essays over and over, hoping the contents will imprint itself on my memory – and block out Mum's voice.

"I can't even go to my own daughter's wedding!" she says, waving a letter written on Doris's personalised letterhead. My sister Julie is getting married and Mum and I are not invited, the letter advises curtly. Doris will be Mother of the Bride. Lorraine is not to come near.

The letter is a double blow: firstly, because Julie doesn't tell us herself, and secondly, because attending isn't an option. The letter prompts a familiar tirade about Julie's allegiance with Dad. I wonder if my sister agreed to Doris's request to be Mother of the Bride to deliberately provoke Mum, in the same way she tried to provoke her when we were children.

The idea that my rebellious sister, who is just 14 months older than me, is doing something as conformist as getting married and will soon wear the label "wife", shocks me. Haven't we both witnessed the havoc marriage wreaked on our mother's life?

Marriage is the chief topic of conversation in our flat in Davies Street since Mum's holiday with Jim, which irritates me.

"Why don't you marry Jim and have a good life?" Nanny says, when she arrives in a taxi, reluctantly paid for by Doris.

"He's not my type. He's too boisterous," Mum says.

"Well, drop him and get someone else," Nanny replies.

"Marriage isn't everything," I say, irritated by this constant talk of matrimony.

"It is at your mother's age," Nanny says, and Mum surprises me by saying I'm being selfish and that she hopes I appreciate her sacrifice, which irritates me even more. How can not wanting to get married be selfish, especially if being married results in being left "with nothing and no one?" I'm sick of appreciating her sacrifice. But it's no good saying so. Instead, I write about it afterwards in copious notes, to try to make sense of it.

I wonder if Julie will regret her marriage, just as our mother did. I haven't seen Julie for five years, so I can't ask her why the sister who's never obeyed anyone is suddenly signing up to "love, honour and obey" her boyfriend Peter. I haven't missed her. I don't care that we aren't invited to the wedding She wants to be a wife. I want to be a journalist.

My prim upright handwriting collapses as the next day, in the English exam, I race to reverse my misspent year.

Two weeks later, I am lying on a hospital trolley wearing nothing but my underwear and a gauzy blue hospital cap and gown, about to undergo another test – to prepare me for my first leg operation – when I hear a familiar voice: "Hello, Janey!"

It's my cousin Pip, his black poodle hair hidden under an identical gauzy blue cap. I knew that he worked in radiology but not that he worked at St Vincent's, where I'm being wheeled into an operating theatre to have blue dye injected into my lymphatic system to track its pathway, ready for my first operation to reconnect the lymph glands in my groin with the blood vessels, in the hope of forming new drainage paths.

"Hello," I say, feeling exposed and disconcerted. Despite being in opposite camps, I still feel bound to Pip and his sister Pam by the joyous Christmases we shared as children and the warmth and affection of their late father, Da – and by the events that divided us. I wonder how Pip feels about having my father turn from uncle to stepfather, but before I can speak, he disappears behind a swinging door with the radiology staff, a ghost returning to the past.

Two hours later, Mr O'Brien inspects my leg. The blue dye from the lympho-angiogram begins confidently and then peters out into an amorphous wash. It's not a good sign, but he'll do the bypass anyway.

A week later, I'm resting on the couch with my leg outstretched, a row of tight spidery black stiches in my groin and instructions to wait and see. Mum brings an assembly line of trays loaded with my favourite foods, which I try to resist, while I read all the books I bought with the $50 she gave me for my 18th birthday earlier that year. When I run out of reading, I think about writing. My English teacher Mrs Jans encouraged me to join the Fellowship of Australian Writers. Anyone could join and receive their newsletter full of members' stories and poems and news of competitions.

As I flick through the newsletter, I see an ad for a playwriting competition. I love the theatre, where life is constructed: beginning, middle and happy ending, at least in musicals, the only theatre I've seen. Whenever we can afford it, Mum and I go together. Afterwards I buy the cast recordings and learn them by heart: *No No Nanette*, starring Nancy Hayes, and the famous American dancer Cyd Charisse, and a new Australian production of *Gypsy* at Her Majesty's

Theatre, which stars Clive Hearn, an Australian actor who performed with Mum in Minnie Everett's production of *The Belle of New York* in Mentone in 1950, five years before her marriage. Mum performed the role of "Fi-Fi Fricot – a little Parisienne", singing *When We Are Married*, with its prophetic warning that "love is not all it's cracked up to be".

"Treading the boards" with Minnie and Clive and her time at the National Theatre Opera School qualifies Mum to comment on these shows with authority, although I always hate it when she insists on introducing herself to the conductor and sings along to the overture, making heads turn. She prefers professional shows, as do I, as twice we are asked to leave amateur Gilbert and Sullivan shows because she's laughing so hard that she snorts.

I've never seen a play but at school we studied Brecht's *Mother Courage and Her Children*, and Shakespeare's *Richard III*, famous for the line "Now is the winter of our discontent." Mum and I have just been through our summer of discontent, equally meaty material for a play. I decide to enter the competition.

I rest my typewriter on my knees and list my characters, Lorraine, 48, Jane 18, Nanny, 80. Setting: A two-bedroom flat in Mentone. Time: The present. The words fly onto the page as I write from the many notes I took to make sense of things after The Great Betrayal, and from our later conversations with Nanny about marriage. I call my play *The Triangle*.

"The End," I type and post it. I don't think about it after that. I'm too busy worrying about my HSC results.

Mum is back at work and I'm staying at Jim's holiday house in Silver Leaves Beach on Philip Island when the results arrive at our flat in Davies Street two weeks later. My hand shakes as I call Mum from a phone box in Cowes, the island's township, for the verdict.

"English – 94."

A small exclamation of delight and pride escapes her. Phew. I draw another breath, waiting.

"English Literature – 91." I exhale. Two out of four.

Social studies – 65.

Oh dear.

French – 56.

Oh no.

I do a quick mental calculation: 306 – six points over the required 300. I still have a chance, confirmed a month later when I receive an offer from RMIT for the first-ever Victorian university course for aspiring journalists.

Mum graduates too, with a certificate in secretarial skills from Stott's. I celebrate by giving her a huge card addressed to

"STOTT'S BEST PUPIL

THE WORLD'S NICEST PERSON AND THE MOST LOVING MOMMA (WHICH REMARKABLY ENOUGH HAPPENS TO BE ALL THE ONE PERSON)."

She gives me a card, too, and a little ceramic angel, because I have "an angel on my shoulder", proven by my success.

I only glance briefly at the letters that arrive from *The Age* and *The Herald*, which all begin with "We regret to inform you …" The RMIT course, which is part-time to accommodate those with cadetships, will begin in February. I need a job. I write to all the local and regional newspapers again and get a job typesetting at RMIT Union while I wait for *The Age* and *The Herald* to reject me.

A few weeks later a letter arrives.

"Congratulations!"

I've won equal third place with another contestant in the Fellowship of Australian Writers junior playwriting competition. The play has been returned with the judge's comments – and a cheque for 30 dollars.

I'm thrilled, but not as thrilled as Mum. She demands to read it, rushing into the bedroom with my play and a new packet of Winfield, to savour them together. I wait anxiously, hoping she'll see it as a work of art: nothing personal.

Half an hour later, she emerges looking like I've run her over.

"You've seen things through the eyes of a child," she says, accusingly.

My face burns.

"I'm going to write you a letter. You can go outside while I write it," she says, dismissing me with a hurt look.

My heart is a slow remorseful thump as I walk slowly around the block.

Twenty minutes later, I return. Silently, she hands me an envelope. Silently, I go to my room and open it with trembling hands.

"The moving finger once having writ moves on," it begins, "Nor all thy piety nor wit can lure it back to cancel half a line."

In brackets underneath is the name Omar Khayyam.

What does it mean? The only thing I understand is the final line: "You must promise NEVER to write anything about me again."

11

The editor slams his fist on his desk: "Even if they fell on the food like a pack of locusts, YOU DON'T WRITE THAT!" he thunders.

I stare, speechless. I finally have a job as a cadet journalist and I'm about to lose it.

After two years of writing to them, begging for a cadetship, Standard Newspapers, in Park Road Cheltenham, has hired me. Hired is the formal term, let loose is the reality. In the full-page report of the Mayoral Ball, the highlight of the municipal social calendar, I gleefully wrote that "a lady took the stool at the piano and plonkety-plonked her way through the same plonkety-plonk tune dozens of times until the last of the 16 deb sets plonked their way down the hall".

With 10 newspapers to oversee, Murray Smith, the news editor, is too busy to edit all our stories BEFORE they're published. His red biro corrections appear on my uncensored stories AFTER publication. Murray grins when complaints pour in, taking it as a sign of reader engagement. I cling to the few letters that are supportive, including one from my former English teacher, Mrs Jans, who declares my report "delightful, entertaining and refreshing".

Tom Young, the editor in chief, whom I'm facing off with in his office, orders an apology, which I do in the form of a poorly drawn cartoon of me as Cinderella being booted out of the Chelsea Town Hall at midnight – prompting another round of complaints.

My slap-dash cartoons, which vaguely imitate Tandberg, the much-loved cartoonist at *The Age*, are championed by Murray and accompany nearly every story I write. I can't help it. I've loved comics and cartoons ever since a neighbour gave me a box of Disney comics when I was bedbound with the mumps at the age of nine, although my drawing skills are no match for my jokes.

I'm scared of losing my job, but not really contrite. I've never been to a debutante ball and find these pretend brides ridiculous. At work, I sit opposite Pola Beran, platinum blonde and buxom, a self-confessed lesbian feminist who writes a weekly column about what real women want: liberation.

It's 1976, one year after The Year of the Woman. In this New World Order women aren't simpering debutants. Nor do they sit around all day complaining about their former husbands. Women have equal pay, health centres, refuges and even a "women's adviser" in the new Government of Prime Minister Malcolm Fraser, a post held by our local MP Ian Macphee, whom I interview regularly without ever questioning why a woman doesn't hold this post. Along with my reports of golden weddings and council meetings, I write a lengthy feature story condemning the profusion of miniature pink vacuum cleaners and ironing boards aimed at little girls in the local toyshop catalogue. Long the champion of one woman, I'm now the champion of all.

"If you ask me, all this women's liberation stuff just liberates men," Mum grumbles, as we do the dishes together after dinner in our flat at Davies Street. Strangely, she never recognises that these reforms also liberate her, as the Whitlam Government allows divorced women to claim the "widow's pension", and grants her a no-fault divorce from Dad, as well as the opportunity to retrain under the National Employment Education and Training Scheme, earning her a job at the newly opened Medibank office in Cheltenham. A husband is now an option rather than a necessity, although husbands are still a good idea.

"At least you had a husband and a family to look after you," Mum reminds Nanny bitterly, as they sit drinking sherries together on her monthly visit. "At least you were protected. You were so protected. You still are. I got no protection. I never did."

I begin to wish Mum would seek protection from Jim and live happily ever after with him in Brighton, leaving me free to stay over at Danny's place.

Danny is the official photographer and my partner in crime at the Chelsea Mayoral Ball, earning similar complaints for his photo of the Mayor with his mouth open – mid fork. We met at Learning Exchange, the community newspaper in East Malvern, where, on Dale's advice, I volunteered for experience to help me get a cadetship, and where Danny has a job writing and taking photos and supervising the many volunteers who help lay out the paper once a month. The Learning Exchange is based on the notion that knowledge can be bartered. It began as a monthly listing of "I want to learn" and "I want to teach" advertisements and morphed into a community newspaper.

Between living at Davies Street with Mum, working as a cadet journalist at Standard News and studying journalism part-time at RMIT, I spend my weekends at Danny's place in Canterbury, returning in the early hours of Monday morning behind the weary clop of the milkman's horse as Danny drives me home.

Danny is 25, six years older than me, with rich dark curly hair worn Afro-style, slim with a pixie face and a black moustache and one of those beards that grows more under the chin than on the face. He wears the body-hugging shirts that are the fashion, smokes Marlborough cigarettes, reads *Esquire Magazine* and *Rolling Stone*, and beats time on his broken steering wheel, singing *Love Potion No. 9* as we drive along in his old yellow Volkswagen.

Danny isn't "comfortable", according to Mum's measure of security. His salary is half a seconded teacher's wage, shared by Kerry, who founded The Learning Exchange with her husband John. But I'm comfortable with him. Our shared interest in newspapers and social issues puts us on common ground.

Nothing has changed in my leg since the operation to bypass the dysfunctional lymph glands in my groin, except I have a jagged raised scar. I'm disappointed but not surprised. Hadn't Mum always said nothing could be done? My surgeon, Mr O'Brien, is disappointed too and offers to sculpt a new leg by removing the hard fibrotic lymphatic tissue. But I'm not ready. I have a new job and a new boyfriend who, like Dale, doesn't comment on my leg, and a new future. I also have plans – although I don't mention them to Mum.

Three months before the Chelsea Mayoral Ball, on a cold winter night after a busy production weekend, Danny put a fresh piece of paper in the old green metal Remington typewriter at Learning Exchange and typed the question he couldn't ask – perhaps we could live together?

Living together would be "sort of" like being married. Can you stand me enough for that? I know I CAN.

I could too. We agreed to move out with friends as soon as we'd saved more money.

I don't want to get married; I just want to get away. My mother's relentless need for reassurance about life, work and Jim is wearing me down.

"And you like them?" she asks, her eyebrow arched inquisitorially above her glassy green eyes, when she asks about Danny's job and family. She never comments on the answers. This is disconcerting. My mother is a woman of strong opinions: she loves the colour red, she "loathes" small talk, she loves prawns, she loathes "toe covers", her word for the useless things sold in gift shops. Yet, she offers no opinion about any of my boyfriends. In her silence, I feel her disapproval, but I dare not ask her opinion directly, for fear of having it confirmed.

A few months later, Danny takes me to meet his family. His mother Shirley greets us at the front door of the neat brick house in Blackburn, wearing a pretty floral apron. Danny has spoken so often about Shirley, whom he calls by her name, that I like her already.

She has the same pixie face, full puckered lips and curly hair as Danny, except she went white at 30 and her hair forms soft meringue peaks around her face. Her figure is soft and womanly and she wears no make-up, apart from pink lipstick.

Danny's blushing 14-year-old brother Michael sits opposite me at the sleek teak dining table, flashing a metallic smile. Their father Howard, a short man with Menzies-like bushy black eyebrows, glows as he tells us how he managed to reach Ecuador on his short-wave radio, while Shirley serves us roast lamb and gravy with freshly shelled peas and home-made mint sauce in a little sauce boat. We talk about Danny's work and my work and Danny's two married sisters, Liz and Jenny and their children. I tell them Mum is divorced. It's just the two of us, which is fine.

A few weeks later, Shirley invites me for afternoon tea. Freshly baked butterfly cakes, garnished with strawberry jam, whipped cream and a gentle dusting of icing sugar, sit on a pretty blue-and-white plate on the dining table beside a tiny crystal vase of dewy violets. The violets remind me of Kathryn Grayson's wedding bouquet of pink rosebuds and violets in the musical *Kiss Me Kate*. The butterfly cakes remind me of Nanny, resting her cream china mixing-bowl between her knees in Florence Street as she whips butter and sugar with an ancient wooden spoon for similar fairy cakes when I am a child. And Shirley's conversation reminds me of … well, I have nothing to compare it to.

"I went down to Lizzy's to see the children, and we had a very happy day," she says, talking about her eldest daughter and her two little girls. Lizzy and her husband Rodger have bought a "dear little house" at Inverloch, which Shirley is looking forward to seeing.

She shows me around her own house, commenting that she's been so busy studying for her diploma as a library technician that she still hasn't made the curtains for her daffodil yellow kitchen or the two bedspreads she plans to sew for the bedrooms. "The material has been here for months", she says, but she'll soon get to it. She's had a visit from her sister Marjorie, whom she hasn't seen for weeks, and they "leaned on the table for hours, catching up". Marjorie is a marvellous dressmaker, and Shirley describes with beaming admiration the wonderful outfits she sews for her many grandchildren.

With intriguing sympathy, she tells me how "poor Howard", Danny's father, went to war after they married and came home to the two children who'd grown in his absence, and whom he hardly knew. Danny and his little brother Michael were born after the war and Howard supported the family as a furniture salesman.

"He still can't help turning every bit of furniture he sees upside down to see how it's made," Shirley says, smiling.

Fathers who work at one job and support their families, sisters who admire each other and talk for hours, mothers who bake and sew. Who could ask for anything more?

"The violets are beautiful," I say, as I rise to leave.

"Come out to the garden and I'll pick you some before you go," Shirley says, leading me out to the back yard she's planted and tended, and where violets grow in moist dark soil, warmed by a quilt of tanbark, amid luminous unfurling tree ferns, replicating in miniature the mystical forests in the Dandenong Ranges. I wave goodbye to Shirley inhaling the intoxicating smell of domestic harmony.

"You're spending a lot of time at Danny's parents' place," Mum observes over dinner one night. I know what's coming.

"And you like them?" she says, her eyebrow arching. Of course, I like them. What's not to like? Shirley never asks whether I like people. Once, she confessed that when an unexpected visitor dropped in for tea, she cut herself a fake chop from a thick slice of white bread and fried that, to save the visitor the embarrassment of knowing there weren't enough chops to go around.

The conversation at our place has turned once again to marriage. My cousin Julianna, Aunt Iris's daughter, is getting married. Amazingly, Mum and I are invited to the wedding, as Doris and Dad are away, and we are going, even though Mum says my cousin is "marrying beneath her".

"He took her to the dogs!" Mum says. "The dogs" is greyhound racing, where no one of refinement goes.

The invitation is to "Lorraine and friend", but Mum doesn't want to subject Jim to that much scrutiny, so I go as "friend".

Mum and I stand at the back of the big bluestone church in Doncaster, away from the curious gaze of the family members that we haven't seen for four years, and watch as my beautiful cousin Julianna with the two "n"s, walks down the aisle in a dazzling white satin dress. I don't know why we're there. Perhaps it's in defiance of Doris's ban on Mum and I attending my sister Julie's wedding the previous year, but it's a discomfiting experience to be strangers amongst family. We don't go "afterwards at the Windsor Hotel", as the invitation offers.

Later that night at home, Mum tells me the groom's father boasted that his son was "marrying into money". These relentless criticisms feel ungenerous and irritate me. It irritates me too, when she insists on vacuuming around me and singing as I clip my stories from that week's *Moorabbin Standard* or *Mordialloc Chelsea News* and paste them in my scrapbook.

"You can't stand to see me having fun, can you?" she says, stopping the vacuum cleaner and staring at me accusingly.

"I'm trying to read," I yell, retreating to my room and slamming the door. The next day is Friday, and Mum is getting ready to go out with Jim, complaining about how she can't stand the "small talk" of "the Brighton crowd", who are his friends.

"If you don't like 'those people', don't go," I say.

"You don't understand," she says. "Who else would have a woman on her own, with nothing and no one? You can't just walk into someone else's situation and give nothing in return."

That night, she comes home late, flushed and swaying, smelling of alcohol.

"I'm a bit the worse for wear, aren't I?" she says, sheepishly.

I've never seen anyone in my family drunk before. The Cafarellas are famous for falling asleep after one drink and the Hills are famous for staying upright after six. As I help her into bed, tugging her slimline white trousers over her big puffy feet, she begins to cry.

"You never complain," she says, staring at me with a strange intensity.

"About what?"

"Your leg … anything," she says, her mascara-streaked tears creating clown-like lines down her cheeks.

I am surprised and touched. She's seen into my soul in a way I hadn't thought possible. I don't complain because there's no point. Nothing can be done about my leg. Hasn't the failed operation proven it? And what's the point of complaining to Mum, who's already wounded?

"It's all right. Sweet dreams! Sleep tight! Hope the bed bugs don't bite," I chime.

Instead, I complain to Danny, who comes to the rescue in his purring yellow Volkswagen beetle.

"What are your plans?" Mum asks one night. "Are you happy staying here?"

"Of course."

How can I move out? The echo of her familiar lament, "Here I am at the age of 47 (now 48,) with nothing and no one" hangs in the air. At the same time, she begins to tell me, "Always have something of your own", as a kind of warning to guard my independence. I do have something of my own – my job – but I need more. I need a proper family, with cakes and violets, not complaints and regrets.

A few weeks later on the way to a meeting at 3CR, the left-leaning community radio station Danny is writing about for Learning Exchange, he pulls over and turns to face me.

"Will you marry me?" he blurts.

"Yes," I say, and we drove on to the meeting, casting shy glances at each other.

"We're engaged," we confess as the meeting ends, receiving a hearty round of applause.

I expect no such applause from Mum. I'm abandoning her to the fate she's so often lamented – being alone with nothing and no one – yet she says nothing when we tell her, except "congratulations".

"Thank you, Lorraine," Danny says, reaching for his packet of Marlborough and offering her a cigarette, and he promises to take good care of me.

I'd have one too, if I smoked.

Just as she sees no future for herself with Jim, I know she sees no future for me with Danny. With no further funding, a wage rise at Learning Exchange is unlikely and he has no formal qualifications. He left his previous job in the office of a toilet paper factory because he hated it. He only ended up at Learning Exchange because the place where he initially chose to offer himself as a volunteer was closed that day.

But in my heart, I know it's not Danny Mum expects great things from. It's me. It's up to me to achieve "something of my own" to make all her sacrifice worthwhile – not to marry a no-hoper who can't "provide".

I don't care. I'll provide for myself. I will have "something of my own", with my own dreams – and a family where no one expects me to make them feel better.

12

The only part my mother takes in the wedding preparations is to meet Shirley to discuss the menu. She doesn't say she won't take part in the other preparations. She just doesn't offer, or maybe she does and in my defensive state, I decline? Either way, I shop alone for a wedding dress, taking the train to the city one Saturday morning, where I choose a Victorian-style cream antique lace three-quarter length dress with ruffled, three-quarter sleeves, which I wear over a long cream satin skirt that Gail's mother makes – and white Homypeds. Neither Danny nor I contemplate a church wedding. I don't want to be a traditional bride, the type I lampooned in my report of the Chelsea debutante ball. I find the celebrant myself – one of my lecturers at RMIT who has a wedding business on the side.

When Shirley suggests we marry in the violet-strewn miniature rainforest in her backyard, with a buffet dinner afterwards, I happily agree. I know Mum can't afford a formal wedding reception and I don't want one anyway. For Christmas that year, Danny gives me a small cookbook to go with the crockpot my mother gives me. The recipe for happiness.

I don't feel the absence of my mother's support. I don't know any better. I've only been to two weddings – my cousin Pam's when I was 12, and my cousin Julianna's the previous year. I know nothing of the organisational rituals. If Mum had insisted on being involved, if we'd spent time together talking invitations, dresses and cakes, we would also talk husbands, which I'm anxious to avoid. The only observation she makes is about the ring, a modest solitaire in platinum gold, rather than the traditional yellow gold.

"It's like you don't mean it," she says, hinting at a deeper truth.

Danny is kind and I love him, but I'm not in love or lust with him. If either of us looked we would have seen that. Once, when we argue, he writes me an apologetic letter suggesting that in future we should aim for "a shared mutuality of expectations", but we never discuss what these expectations may be.

Two weeks before the wedding he writes me another letter with his favourite Osmoroid pen telling me "what a fine person" I am, and how lucky he feels. He's a fine person, too: finer than me. Throughout our courtship I've been having a secret affair with Leon, my work colleague, with whom I share a passion for theatre and the occasional midnight dalliance in the Frankston office. Leon never tries to dissuade me from marrying Danny. He seems to accept that our affair will end after the wedding, as do I. He even enlists his aunt to make my wedding cake. Torn between my need for family and security and my need to break free, I am hedging my bets, building myself a corral, while happily jumping over it whenever it suits.

"Have you been practising your new signature?" the girl at the print shop says when I go to pick up the wedding invitations.

"What new signature?"

"For your new name."

"I'm not changing my name," I say firmly.

I choose a husband and wedding invitations without ever considering I'm choosing a new identity.

Yet, I never imagine *not* marrying Danny.

"You *are* getting married, aren't you?" the real estate agent asks as we sat opposite him, poised to sign the papers for our new home – a modest one-bedroom flat in Bourke Street, Mentone. Along with one month's rent in advance, it seems another bond is required.

"Of course," I reply.

I don't feel my father's absence in the wedding preparations either. We've had no contact since the day Mum found out about his affair with Doris. Our relationship doesn't exist and neither does he. Nor does my sister Julie. She chose Doris as Mother of the Bride for her own wedding – without inviting Mum or me. It feels natural, even right, not to invite her to mine. I hardly know the guests from Danny's side of the family. My cousin Pip will bring Nanny, the only guest from Mum's side. The only people invited from Dad's side are his youngest sisters Tess and Tina, whom I haven't seen since the Great Betrayal. Tess and Tina are like Switzerland: neutral, perhaps even allies. Whenever they visited us in Remo Street, Dad put on the record of the Stripper, and Julie and I watched pop-eyed as trumpets as rude as farts sounded and Tess, Tina and Mum rose in an unspoken pact and writhed sensually around the room, transformed.

The night before the wedding, Mum watches as I lay out my dress, ready to take it to Shirley's after a visit to the hairdresser, where I will be transformed from girlfriend to wife.

"You don't have to do this," she says quietly.

"I want to," I say, and I do. I want to be free from this game where she's the perpetual victim and I'm her saviour. She doesn't raise it again.

On the day of the wedding, which is also Danny's 26th birthday, Gail helps secure the white tuber roses in my hair, which are piled elegantly on my head, and carrying a small bouquet of white gardenias and yellow rose buds I step into Shirley's lounge room where the celebrant and a small group of guests are waiting.

I gaze at Danny's burgundy velvet suit and matching bow tie in astonishment. "It was the only suit left at the hire place," he whispers. I hadn't realised it was traditional for the bride to also choose the groom's outfit.

The next morning the burgundy suit is replaced by Danny's familiar sunflower yellow bathrobe, tied with an old school tie, as he stands before me bearing a plate of bacon and matching sunflower-yellow eggs at the holiday house in Inverloch his sister has lent us for our honeymoon. I sit up in bed, trying to look grateful. I feel a bit queasy and put it down to the runny eggs and the cold I feel coming on.

Later that day, we go exploring, but with every curve in the road, my queasiness increases. I'm not hungry the next morning either. By the third morning, neither of us has any appetite as the local doctor at Inverloch leans back in his chair.

"Congratulations!" he beams.

***

There was no carelessness on my part. The pregnancy was the result of a failed IUD. The doctor at Mentone I'd consulted the previous year refused to give me the pill due to my mother's history of thrombosis, as it increased the risk of blood clots. I didn't want a baby. I was only one year into my cadetship. Mr O'Brien was planning the first big reduction operation on my leg later that year. A year earlier, I'd politely declined Danny's youngest sister's invitation to hold her pink and squirming new-born infant. Hadn't my mother always warned me that babies were a nuisance and a trap?

As soon as we return from our honeymoon Danny accompanies me to the euphemistically named Fertility Control Clinic in Wellington Parade East Melbourne. We leave two hours later – liberated. We don't tell anyone. It's none of their business. Nor do we speak of it again, not because we're ashamed but because it's no longer relevant. It doesn't occur to me the baby might have been Leon's. In my mind, my only real relationship was with my prospective husband.

Relieved, we throw ourselves into our work – endless meetings and long weekends of laying out the paper for Danny and a new position as a junior reporter on *The Moorabbin Standard* for me. Feminism is bubbling up all around me and I'm diving in, with a front-page story about "domestic" violence and a headline that screams, "Women need refuge", while at home at weekends I do the shopping and the housework. Most Sundays we visit Shirley and Howard for a

Sunday roast, or listen to Danny's favourite program on radio station 3CR, *Nostalgia Unlimited*, featuring music from the 1920s, 30s and 40s – while I do the ironing on a bigger version of the pink ironing boards I wrote about so scathingly two years earlier.

The world of the Gigolo and the Monster and my mother's pain feels far away. It's no longer The Ma and the Kid, it's Danny and Jane. Only occasionally, by arrangement, does Mum visit, always fashionably dressed and heavily made up, bearing sherry and flowers. I don't miss her. I'm enjoying my new life – taking risks at work if not at home, egged on by my new boss George Coote, who signs himself George the Red, and who specialises in subversion.

During the long Christmas break, I have the first of the four operations to reduce and sculpt my leg. The operation involves slicing off the fibrotic lymphatic tissue on the inside of my leg from mid-thigh to ankle. The result is revealed to me a week later when the nurse changes the dressing in Mr O'Brien's rooms as he inspects his handiwork. I look like the victim of shark attack. My knee looks like it's shifted to the left and a saw-toothed track of black bloody stitches run from the outside of my leg down my calf in a jagged line down the centre of the pillow of flesh on the top of my foot, now only slightly deflated. My leg buzzes, sizzles and aches, but I don't care.

"I'm thrilled to bits," I tell my colleagues in a four-page comic-book style letter sent back with my boss Murray, who visits every Wednesday with my pay packet. Until then, I've avoided questions about why I wear long dresses, deflecting their gaze with jewellery and fitted tops.

After two weeks in hospital, I am discharged with crutches and a pink elastic tubi-grip compression stocking into Mum's care at our old apartment in Davies Street, as Danny's long hours mean he won't be home until late each night.

One day Mum comes in shuffling the contents of the mailbox. "This is for you," she says, handing me an envelope. For me? Since my marriage, all my mail has gone to the flat I share with Danny in Bourke Street, Mentone.

I tear it open. "Best wishes for your recovery." Inside, in tiny ant-like writing, is the message: "Glad to hear the operation was a success – Julie and Peter XXX." Get well wishes from my sister and her husband.

I'm surprised and touched, although the card says nothing about her life and asks nothing about mine.

"Nanny must have told her," Mum says

I don't hear from my father, nor do I expect to. I return home to Danny and to work.

A month later, the shrill alarm of the phone interrupts my ironing and the scratchy warblings on *Nostalgia Unlimited*.

The voice on the phone is rich and resonant. I recognise it instantly as belonging to my cousin Kathy – Aunty Mary's daughter – although I haven't seen her since we were teenagers.

"Uncle Frank's had an accident," she says.

Uncle Frank? It takes a moment to register that Uncle Frank is my father. I haven't heard anyone refer to him as Uncle Frank for years, as I'm no longer in touch with any of my cousins on Dad's side of the family. I listen as Kathy tells me how earlier that night "Uncle Frank" arrived in an ambulance at the Emergency Department at St Vincent's Hospital, where she works as a nurse. He was working night shift at a factory when he leaned on a machine, which he thought was turned off. The machine whirred into action, severing all four fingers on his left hand.

I wish she'd said he was dead. Whatever he wasn't, my father was a man of imagination, creativity and invention, always making and doing, even if seldom finishing. What would he make and do now? Who cared if he never pays the bills? Who cared that he ran off with my mother's sister? Of course, I would go and see him.

I scan the faces of the men as I walk through the Spartan men's ward at St Vincent's public hospital, so different from St Vincent's Private next door, where I'd had my own operation, and where a glass of wine was offered with every meal. It's three years since I've seen my father. I've grown up. I have a job and a husband. How will we great each other – as father and child, or equals?

"It's good to see you, love," he says, when I finally find him, dressed in blue-striped flannelette pyjamas. He looks older but his blue eyes are as frightened as a child's as he holds up the bandaged fist of his left hand in a fingerless salute.

He recounts the story of the accident. Someone scooped up the fingers in the hope that a skilful surgeon might magically restore them. At the Emergency Department, my cousin Kathy appeared like an angel to sooth and salve. Then came the crushing news from the doctors: there would be no miracle. The fingers couldn't be reattached. Finally, the resignation: this was his new identity, his new story, to be added to the lexicon of mythic and tragic tales my family seemed to live by.

He throws back the bed covers, to show me the other half of the story – the flesh that's been scooped from his thigh and grafted over the place where his fingers once were. They're going to operate again later to create a pincer from the remains of his left thumb, he says. He was working under a false name, so claiming Worker's Compensation is complicated.

"How's your mother?" he asks when he finally draws breath, as if he's asking fondly about an old friend.

"Fine," I say. I'm fine. She's fine. What else can we be in the face of such tragedy? He pauses.

"You're married now," he says, his eyes landing on my own left hand with its five intact fingers and the wedding and engagement rings on the fourth. Nanny and Pip told him all about it.

"I was going to get a video camera and film it," he says, with a flash of familiar bravado.

"How?"

"Round the back, through the fence."

I gaze at him in surprise. It never occurred to me that he might want to come to my wedding: that he felt entitled to come. Didn't he realise he'd forfeited that right by divorcing me along with my mother? I have a new family now. I'm visiting him because I feel sorry for him, not because I want to reinstate him.

"Anyway, Dad … " I say, rising to leave.

"By the way," he says, suddenly animated. "The guitar's no use to me now. Do you want it?"

I stop. Do I want the Holy Grail of my childhood, the cup of happiness my sister and drank from in those rare moments of harmony in Remo Street when we were children? Of course I want it, and he promises to send it to me.

* * *

Mum tries to be magnanimous when I tell her about the accident when we meet in a cafe in the city a few days later. "I'm very sorry to hear that," she says.

She pauses, sips her coffee, and looks up: "I'll bet Doris won't want him now."

It's the suggestion that I might visit him again to pick up the guitar that really upsets her.

"It's your decision," she says with pursed lips.

"It's not a decision. I'm just going to get the guitar."

"Let's change the subject."

"He is my father," I say, annoyed by the assumption I've crossed a line.

She cocks her head and looks at me with flinty eyes. "He wasn't a father's bootlace." And as if to test my loyalty, she says, "You know I can wipe you, just as I wiped that Monster and Julie."

A chill comes over me, but before I can react, she says, "You're very irritable lately. Everything all right between you and Danny?"

I recognise it as deflection. She's responding to what she sees as my threat of abandonment with a threat of her own. I don't contact my father again, nor does he contact me. Instead, he sends the guitar.

Like my relationship with my father, it's broken. The blonde spruce top is paper-thin; there's green paint on the back and a crack on the side and no case.

"You can have any guitar in the shop if you leave it here," the shop assistant says when I take it to my local music shop to inquire about repairs. If he wants it that badly, then I do too. I take it home and look up "guitar repair" in the *Yellow Pages*.

The young man with the medieval sounding title of "luthier" examines it with the same focus Mr O'Brien examined my leg on my first visit, running his hand gently over the dull wood. It's a 1926 Martin parlour guitar, made in Nazareth, Pennsylvania, USA, he tells me. "Worth a bit of money, but not playable, not in this condition."

Worth less if he fixes it, but at least I can play it. I choose to play it.

Mum doesn't ask about it, or whether I'm seeing my father. She's finally broken up with Jim. He moved to Hobart for work, and in a last-ditch attempt to persuade her to marry him, he invited her there to see if she liked it. She didn't and left a few days later as the sole passenger on a midnight flight, where she was invited to sit in the cockpit with the captain.

Shortly afterwards, on a chilly Saturday morning, I answer the front door of our flat in Bourke Street to a stranger.

"Your mother's not well," he says, introducing himself as Tony, Mum's new boyfriend. She's in hospital. The thrombotic vein in her leg exploded, spattering blood all over the walls and floor of the flat in Davies Street. I'm spattered too – with guilt. I abandoned my mother for marriage and it fell to a stranger to tell me she was in hospital bleeding to death.

"The doctor said it could happen again any time," Mum says, giving me a told-you-so look when I fly to her bedside.

My sister Julie is sick too. Through Nanny we hear she's been throwing up and losing weight. Mum shakes her head, regarding the news as an extension of my sister's refusal to eat as an infant – another example of her perversity. A few weeks later, Nanny rings to say Julie has been diagnosed with diabetes.

"It's all that sugar she ate," Mum says.

I know nothing about diabetes and how serious it is; just that it requires injections. I don't question my mother's interpretation.

I'm throwing up too. The new IUD the doctor insisted upon has proven as useless as the first. Our prospects have only marginally improved. I've been promoted to third-year cadet at Standard News, which means a small pay rise, but Danny is still earning the same wage. We've already upgraded our health insurance to pay for my next operation, planned for the following year. Mr O'Brien has also raised a sobering fact: lymphoedema may be hereditary.

There's no suggestion from Danny that a child with lymphoedema will be rejected. The unease is all on my part. Only I know what it really means to live with a deformity that can't be explained or cured. We make no definitive decision about having children, but the suggestion of inheritance is enough for us to agree to another abortion. It's a convenient out. I had no regrets about the first abortion and have no hesitation about this one. Like daughters throughout time, the limitations of my mother's life have been held up to me like a mirror I'm determined to smash.

So blasé am I about this second "procedure", I stupidly rearrange the furniture in the flat the next day. The day after, I'm visiting my Aunt Tess's for lunch with Mum – our first visit since my wedding. Amid the laughter and the jokes, I begin to feel faint. Before I can say anything, I fall face-first into my soup. I wake on the couch to find Mum, Tess and her sister Tina hovering over me. I try to explain I've had an abortion – and that I've had one before. But my words are garbled. Instead of "before" they mishear and think I said "four" – quadrupling their horror.

Mum is quiet as she drives me home. She fills a vase for the daisies my old paramour Leon left at the door after hearing that I was sick, and tucks me into bed.

"You know, it's okay to have a baby," she says, holding my gaze.

I nod, but I don't believe her. Okay to end up like her? NEVER!

***

The life I want is represented by a small framed picture of a medieval lute player, titled *Le Musicien*, which I buy in a print shop in West Melbourne and place on my old pedal organ, when Danny and I move from the flat in Bourke Street, Mentone, to a two-bedroom art deco-style flat in Bates Street East Malvern, to be closer to Learning Exchange. The picture, a modest print, feels like a talisman that will bring music back into my life. My father's guitar has come back to me, sleek and shiny; the green paint gone, the crack and the fret board repaired and with new metal strings, giving it a richer, brighter tone. I plan to learn – as soon as I find a teacher.

The high ceilings and echoing acoustics of the dark wooden panelling in the new apartment improve my voice, and while Danny's at work I sing all the old songs Mum and Dad sang, and all my favourite songs from musicals, grateful that the downstairs tenant doesn't complain. Publicly, I've always wanted to be a journalist. Privately, I've always wanted to be able to sing just like my mother. At 16, I entered the school talent quest as a solo performer, singing *Second Hand Rose*, which Mum had sung with her own little singing trio when I was a child. I wore a long navy-blue satin dress and long white gloves from the op shop and rehearsed with Gail, who played piano. But on the night, I stood in front of the microphone, sweating in terrified silence, before stumbling through the song.

"You had stage fright," Mum said afterwards, offering no further comment.

Good acoustics and the refurbished guitar give me new hope that I'll overcome stage fright, inspired by the local Green Man Folk Club in East Malvern.

Together with Jenny and John – two of the many volunteers who help out at the Learning Exchange production weekend – Danny and I spend most Saturday nights at The Green Man, which is famous for its pancakes and its music – mostly played by men with guitars. I take more than a casual interest in these guitar-clad men, giving them god-like status as I watch their fingers fly over fret boards and caress strings, their eyes closed in self-absorbed ecstasy.

"Do you teach?" I ask the one I admire the most, and my heart sings when he says yes. Every Wednesday, I drive to Carlton for lessons, but I make little progress, despite my diligent practice. Every man with a guitar is my father and every critic is my mother.

Not that Mum takes much interest. She's too busy with the news she's extracted from Nanny during their weekly phone call. Doris and Dad have married at the registry office, with just Julie, her husband Peter, my cousins Pip and Pam, and Pam's husband and daughter as witnesses. I imagine the wedding photo: Doris and Dad, the bride and groom, flanked by my sister and cousins, in the same way my two grandmothers had flanked Dad and Mum in their wedding photo 22 years earlier. I wonder how my cousins felt about my father – whom they had always known as Uncle Frank – now being their legal stepfather. I guess I'll never know: more than ever, the marriage cements the family division. To mark the occasion, Dad changes his name to Frank Caff, which Nanny thinks is a good thing, since he'll no longer be associated with Mum, who's still Lorraine Cafarella.

"It's because that Monster doesn't want to be the next Mrs Cafarella," Mum says.

I guess he changed his name to change his luck. For Dad, being a Cafarella was a curse, attracting bullying and name-calling as a child for being a "wog" and bad luck as an adult.

For my mother, the marriage makes their betrayal official and complete.

"She must have really hated me," she says, when Nanny tells her the details.

A month later, she extracts more news.

My sister has given birth to a daughter, born early due to the complications of diabetes. I didn't want to be a mother but I didn't count on being an aunty.

"Isn't it disgusting?" Mum says. "My own daughter, and I had to find out like this."

I think of the card Julie sent after my most recent leg operation. "Best wishes for your recovery." I wonder if I should return the gesture. Yet this milestone in my sister's life – the same milestone that I determinedly avoided – seems to deserve something more. I visited Dad in hospital in his hour of need. It feels like the right thing to visit my sister in hers. It also feels like entering the lion's cage. What will she do when she sees me: throw something at me – like talcum powder, hot water or orange juice, as she did when we were children?

Yet there in lingers another memory – "They're fighting again," we whisper to each other as we lay under our paisley pink quilts in Remo Street as children, listening to waves of angry voices. We don't fight. We swap the books our Aunt Ga gives us for Christmas and both fall in love with *The Little White Horse* by Elizabeth Goudge and its heroine, Maria Merryweather, a Moon Princess, whose adventure starts when she becomes an orphan. With the five cents pocket money Mum gives us each week, we save up for a set of six tiny records in a box from the tobacco shop in Mentone Parade as a gift for Mum and Dad. "They're coasters, to put drinks on," the shopkeeper explains. We buy them anyway because they will make Mum and Dad happy.

My heart knocks in time as I knock on the hospital room door.

"Come in," a voice I don't recognise says.

I poke my head around, "It's me, Jane," I say, half in warning.

She looks tired and startled. The birth was sudden, she explains. The baby, a girl, is swaddled in a crib next to her bed, an anonymous parcel whose life and personality are yet to unfold: the easy focus of our conversation.

"She's over her jaundice now," Julie says. "There's nothing wrong with her except she's prem and her lungs aren't working properly."

There's a chance she might have diabetes. "We have to watch her for the first 12 months."

I nod sympathetically, noting how history has repeated itself with another premature daughter. She thanks me for the gift I bring, although I can't recall what it was, just that she mentions in a puzzled voice that our cousin Diana, who'd recently given birth to twins, gave her three pairs of plastic pants, which felt like a warning for all the shit that was in store, rather than congratulations.

"How's Mum?" she says when the talk of babies and husbands is depleted. "Good," I say. "How's Dad?"

"Good," she says.

I search for words to fill the silence that follows, but none come.

"Thanks for coming," she says, and we go back to our separate lives – mine with a new leg and a new job and hers with a new baby.

Mum has a new baby, too. For her 50th birthday the previous April, I gave her what she'd always craved: a Chihuahua puppy. We went together to the breeder to choose it – a spindly, shivery, blonde long-haired puppy called Possum, which Mum carries like a handbag wherever she goes. Possum even goes to work with her in her new job as a receptionist at the Malvern Tennis Centre, shivering on Mum's lap while the well-to-do ladies in tennis whites gush over them both.

When Mum goes away with a friend, I take Possum to work, where she sits in her basket beside my desk, shivering and shaking while my work colleagues gush over her. *The Herald and Weekly Times* has taken over Standard News and the new managing editor has declared our newsroom the worst in the world, sending white-clad masked fumigators to banish the fleas from the carpet, which I'm sure were living there way before Possum turned up for work.

The new manager also orders the removal of all the wall graffiti, including all my cartoons. As compensation, he offers $10 for every cartoon published each week, capped to $50 within the week, after I immediately churn out 10 that week, quickly earning myself an extra hundred dollars.

He's less enamoured with my front-page expose for the Christmas edition of the Sandringham paper that year. As a spoof on the push for nude bathing at Sandringham Beach, I persuaded a male colleague of wide girth to dress as Santa, gradually stripping off as he ran into the gently lapping waves – his Santa hat and boots in the foreground and his bare bottom in the background.

"This is a family newspaper," the new manager says, chastising me. Once more, I'm not contrite. I'm a risk taker. Except on weekends, when I'm a domestic goddess, presiding over dinner parties and learning to sew.

The operations have reduced my leg, as promised, but they've also made it lumpy and misshapen and turned my right foot into a puffy rectangle. The long Indian style skirts I wore to hide my legs in previous years are out of fashion, so I make my own. Sewing doesn't come naturally. Often, I buy the wrong material or choose patterns too complicated for my skills, resulting in secret tears of frustration. I don't want to show my ankles, which are still padded with wads of lymphatic tissue, so the skirts and dresses I make drag along the ground. On wet days, the hems become muddy and soggy and begin to rot, hanging in uneven tatters. On windy days, they cling to my legs, exposing my secret as I struggle down the street. Finally, I give up and go to a local seamstress, but the long dresses and skirts she makes look strange – neither day nor evening wear.

When a red rash appears on my big leg one Sunday morning, accompanied by fever and chills, Danny calls a locum doctor.

"You've got cellulitis," the doctor says. Cellulitis is a bacterial skin infection. The scar tissue from the surgery has made the skin more vulnerable to infection.

"It might be easier just to have the leg amputated," he says casually as he prepares an injection of penicillin. I stare at him in silent horror. Over my dead body.

13

I not only keep my leg, I improve it. Six months later, in the second operation to reduce it, Mr O'Brien slices the outside to match the inside, sculpting it into a new slimmer shape. My new leg rests in a plaster trench lined with cotton wool. A week later, I develop a dull pain in the heel and a temperature.

"Take it off!" Mr O'Brien says tersely to the nurses who hover anxiously. "Yes, Mr O'Brien. Sorry, Mr O'Brien," they chorus as they remove the trench.

The infection means another week in hospital. I don't mind. I'm tired and glad to be in this quiet white world with its predictable and comforting rhythms. The kindly nurses in their crisp white uniforms, freshly showered and perfumed with each new shift, give me a spare IV pole to poke at the TV to change the channel. The congenial catering staff smile as they check my completed menus. The courteous cleaners admire my flowers, and flocks of black-suited doctors from around the world follow Mr O'Brien, keen to learn about this new treatment for lymphoedema, turning both of us into celebrities.

Into this white world, like a splash of red paint on a white wall, comes Mum, charming us all, always in red, with matching red lips and green frosted eyelids, her customary bun softened by a fringe and kiss curls glued in place with hair spray.

"Your mother's very glamorous," a nurse comments when visiting hours are over. "We'll all have to take lessons in *haute couture* from her."

I'm proud – and sad. My mother is a charming visitor with me too: polite and careful. Outside the hospital, our every conversation feels loaded. If I talk about Danny, she tells me about the remarkable achievements of the sons-in-law of friends who are lawyers or doctors – friends she met through work and her new boyfriend, a tall shy man with the grand and quaintly old-fashioned name of Walter. If I talk about my work she sighs and tells me she thought I might "write something someday", meaning a book, not a report about a council meeting. And when, with clumsy fingers and quavering voice, I give in to her pleas to play guitar and sing for her, she sits with elevated eyebrows and asks if I've heard of "bel canto", the classical method of singing she learned as a girl. Every interaction feels like a judgement, and just like my father, I want to flee.

Hearing the nurses praise her makes me feel teary and regretful that we're no longer close. So, I write to tell her what the nurses have said, adding that I'm proud of her, whether she's glamorous or not, but with work and all, I don't seem to get the time to say it.

It's been three years since we stood together in the back pew of the chapel at the Le Pine funeral parlour in Blackburn, suffering the curious looks of family who were now strangers, as we farewelled Nanny, who'd died at age 86. I'd hardly seen Nanny since she came to my wedding, wearing her fox fur and hat and clutching Pip's arm. In her final years, she'd been too ill to visit us and I'd been too self-absorbed to visit her. In her last visits to us in Davies Street, her balance was so bad the taxi drivers had to escort her up the stairs to our front door. "Thank you, Driver," she said royally to the bemused driver, when I met her at the door.

"We chattered away. They're all nice to me you know," she said. "I'd have my life over again. My word, I would!" and she promised to come back as soon as she could after she died, which infuriated Mum, who felt her life had been unbearable the first time around, and who refused to line up for seconds. As the celebrant who pretended to know my irrepressible Nanny droned on, I said "Hoo-roo, Nanny," and vowed to look out for her.

But it's Mum, not Nanny, who seems to be making a comeback. She's moved from Davies Street in Mentone to a half a house in Wimmera Place, St Kilda, where she paints the kitchen cupboards red and sets up red Tiffany-style lamps with black fringed shades on the benches, making it look like a sultry boudoir. Weekends are spent with Walter, who looks a bit like Carey Grant but with none of his grace. His head leads and his body follows stiffly behind, with that awkwardness that comes from growing too quickly as an adolescent and never quite coming to terms with the suddenness of it all. He's an industrial chemist and a pioneer of the plastics industry, and, like Mum, is divorced with two adult daughters. They seem a good match and I soon get used to seeing Mum with Possum on one arm and Walter on the other.

After I recover from the latest operation, I invite them both to lunch at Bates Street, making dishes from my three favourite cook books: "parsleyed eggs in the half shell" from *The Vegetarian Epicure* (boiled eggs sawn in half and filled with the egg mixed with parsley and cream cheese); coq a vin from *The Women's Weekly Cook Book*, and pineapple upside-down cake from my high school Home Economics textbook, *Cookery The Australian Way*. Walter's large doe-like blue eyes are rarely animated, except when it comes to my mother and food. For months afterwards, he raves about the meal, completely won over, although it's Mum I'm trying to win over. I'm uneasy in her presence, which makes me feel guilty and keen to atone.

Occasionally, Shirley invites Mum to a family lunch at Blackburn, and although she's charming to everyone, in that homely atmosphere the glamour so admired by the nurses in the hospital feels inauthentic and embarrassing. It suits me that she's busy with Walter and their plans on weekends, even if Danny and I have no particular plans of our own. Unlike our friends Jenny and John.

Jenny and John are building their own house in the country on a farm and plan to spend a year travelling around Europe. Every moment, thought and cent is garnered towards these mutual goals as they scour the countryside for old bricks, and spend weekends together restoring old furniture and pouring over *Europe on $20 a Day*.

Inspired, I suggest that perhaps Danny and I could save to travel around Europe for a year. He looks alarmed.

"I don't think I could leave my mother for that long," he says.

I'm not surprised. We visit his mother more than we visit mine, and more than we visit any friends. The only travelling we've done are a few short camping trips around country Victoria to indulge Danny's passion for black-and-white photography, or to visit his sisters – but only when he can afford to get his car serviced.

On the weekends when he's busy with Learning Exchange production, I drive to Jenny and John's new farm in the country to help them make their dreams come true, trowelling mortar across the fireplace built from the second-hand bricks they've collected, and admiring the special alcove in the new kitchen, where newly kneaded bread will rise in the morning sun. I'm a city girl, who breathes a sigh of relief every time I turn off the freeway and stop at my first red light – civilisation! But loneliness and wistful envy keeps me going back.

At home I'm frustrated and irritable. The exhausting Learning Exchange production weekends that keep Danny away feel futile when half the papers he delivers to newsagents and milk bars each month are returned unsold. When he's home, he sits at his desk playing on his IBM computer, or writing stories for Learning Exchange, a task requiring endless "ciggies", "cuppas", sharpening of pencils and refilling of his trusty Osmoroid fountain pen.

I have my own paper to lay out, with real readers. After work, I prefer to read, play guitar and watch musicals. Once, he sets me up in the dining room with a quilt and a glass of wine while I watch *Seven Brides for Seven Brothers*, about a backwoods clan of brothers in Oregon who kidnap their girlfriends so they can marry them. As I watch, Danny checks in on me every half hour with puzzled bemusement, which annoys me. We seem to share nothing but the apartment and a mutual love of Shirley.

"What's wrong?" he asks, looking hurt and confused, while I sulk and slam doors. I'm too ashamed to admit the cocoon I've spun for myself feels constricting. Alone, I play my guitar and sing *Single Girl*, the lament of the girl who regrets her marriage, which my unhappy mother sang – the truth of it echoing in my ears, just as it echoed in hers.

Late one Sunday afternoon after Danny and I argue, I pile some spare bedding and my toiletries into my green VW Beetle and turn up on Mum's doorstep in Wimmera Place St Kilda, tearful and angry. There's nowhere else to go. I don't dare admit to Shirley that I'm unhappy and Jenny and John live too far away for me to stay. Nor do I feel comfortable confiding in them. Previous admissions have felt more useful to them in reinforcing the perfection of their own marriage.

"You can't stay here," Mum says, appearing at the door with Possum in her arms and Walter shadowing her. Feeling foolish, I go home, promising to call later to tell her everything is all right.

Everything is all right – as long as I have some distraction.

"That new guy gave you a lascivious look," a work colleague tells me one day, as we walk out together to buy some lunch.

"What's lascivious?"

"Lustful."

The new guy is Tom, an Irish photographer on a working holiday from Dublin. Tom has unruly black hair, aqua eyes and a tendency to break out into song after one drink. I soon find Tom's name written next to mine whenever I request a photographer. Tom is fun, when I can understand what he says. "Dat's in the Nort," he says dismissively when I ask him about "the Troubles".

One day, instead of going back to the office we go out for a drink.

"Ay, you're a tall gal," he coos as he straddles me in the back of the station wagon on the lonely country road where we divert on the way home. He seems unbothered by my long dress and my compression stocking.

I'm like Sara Monday in *The Horse's Mouth,* my favourite HSC text – "who could commit adultery and weep over it and enjoy both operations at the same time".

I'm not the only one playing around. Some jokester in our office writes "on air' on the small glass window on the swinging door between the two newsrooms at Standard News, and someone else crosses it out and writes "on heat".

I decide I'm way too young to be married. At lunch times I sit complaining to a colleague about the husband I no longer want, without admitting I don't have the courage to leave his family. Instead, I leave my job – and get a new one as General Reporter at *The Herald* in Flinders Street, where I specialise in sob stories.

"A mother wept today …" seems to be my stock story "intro". At the end of the year, my new colleagues award me a box of tissues and I'm promoted to Local Government Reporter.

Eighteen months later, I have the final operation to reduce my leg. Mr O'Brien has come up with a drastic plan. Instead of doing four operations as planned, in the third and final operation he removes everything from the knee down except the muscle and the bone.

My skin rests in a fridge overnight, while my leg lies like a skinless frankfurter swathed in paraffin-soaked bandages in yet another plaster trench padded with cotton wool. The next day, the skin is grafted back on to my slimmer leg, where it will act as a natural compression stocking, as there'll be no space for the lymph to return.

When it's unveiled, I proudly hold up my leg, chorus-girl style, while the nurse takes a photo with a Polaroid. From the knee down it's a bloody mess. I'm more interested in the shape. My right calf looks almost the same size as my left. My foot is still a giant rectangle, but the top is flat, making it so much easier to fit a shoe. I don't care that my lower leg looks like raw meat. I don't care that it turns a magnificent magenta and throbs the first time I try to put it to the ground, and that I have to learn to walk again. I don't care that I look like a burns victim. Burns are normal.

What isn't normal is the sky, which is a dull orange as the acrid smell of smoke fills the room. It's another burning hot day in what's been a mercilessly hot summer. I'm tethered to my bed by fat bags of crimson blood, saline and antibiotics hanging from the metal pole above me.

"The hospital is on fire!" I call in alarm, to the nurse who responds to my urgent buzzing.

"It's just a dust storm," she says.

The next week, temperatures reach 43 Celsius and a fierce dry wind-change sweeps through South Australia and Victoria. Houses explode, possessions and dreams melt and 75 people die. Through Aunty Iris we hear that Dad and Doris were nearly among them, and their new house in Fairhaven, that Dad built with his one-and-a-half hands, has been razed.

"Ha!" Mum says, her eyes glinting. Divine retribution.

I'm sorry about my father's house, and glad he's not dead. But I feel nothing more. We haven't seen each other in six years – not since I visited him in hospital after his fingers were severed. He feels like a character in a movie I once saw. So does my sister. There is no get-well card from my sister for this recent leg operation, either. I doubt she even knows about it. Since Nanny's death, there's no regular news from Camp Dad and Doris.

Three weeks later, I'm discharged home to our flat in Bates Street, in a wheelchair with my leg sticking out on a board in front to keep it elevated. At home, there are no nurses, no cleaners, and no menus to tick off. Everyone is at work, including Danny. Tom, the Irish photographer has long gone back to Ireland and his girlfriend. Mum is still working part-time at the Malvern Tennis Centre and is living with Walter in his bachelor pad in Milton Street, Elwood, where she cooks and he eats. I'm too weak to feel like reading or singing or playing the guitar. I struggle to manoeuvre myself around the flat in the wheelchair, frustrated and bored. The only time I leave is in the back of a taxi with my leg stretched out on the seat, my crutches resting beside me, to go to Mr O'Brien's rooms in East Melbourne to have the dressings changed on the wounds that refuse to heal.

I begin to resent Danny for not taking time off to look after me: for not taking time off work to do anything. Unlike Jenny and John's life, ours is stuck on repeat.

"What do you want to do?" Danny asks on the weekend, as I sit surly and sad in my wheelchair. I want the "shared mutuality of expectations" that he so eloquently described in his letter to me before we married and which we never discussed – although I can't articulate it.

"I want to go to the beach," I say. It's a ridiculous request. I'm still bandaged. I can't walk properly let alone swim. Danny pushes me glumly beside the sea wall, as sunbakers and swimmers frolic by the shore.

I'm not surprised when my old school friend Gail tells me that she cooked a meal for Danny while I was still in hospital, offering herself as a dessert – and that he nervously accepted. She gives me an evaluation of his performance (poor). I don't confront Danny about it. Gail isn't in love with Danny. She's in love with the ex-Hari Krishna, Matthew, whom she later marries. I'm not in love with Danny either. I'm in love with his mother and family.

The days drag as my leg fails to heal.

"You've got Golden Staph," the nurse in Mr O'Brien's rooms whispers one day, as she places a cotton swab soaked in paraffin over the crimson crater on my shin. "You got it in hospital, but they didn't tell you."

Eventually, with mountains of antibiotics, it heals, although these scars are raised and knotted, forming deep trenches on the top of my foot.

"Keloid," the nurse says, explaining that dark-skinned people are more prone to these hard growths. The raised scars are kept flat by the thick compression stockings I must wear for the rest of my life to maintain the shape of my new leg.

As soon as I recover, I go back to my guitar teacher. I'm disappointed when he hands me the phone number of a new teacher, explaining that he is going away for a month. I'm nervous about playing in front of someone new, but I've missed so many lessons already, I can't afford to miss more.

The new teacher's name is Hendrik, which he explains is Dutch, although he prefers Rik. Tall with fine blonde hair and a thick reddish-blond beard, he is softly spoken, guarded, a little awkward and … sad. The room where he sleeps and gives guitar lessons contains nothing but a mattress on the floor, a sheet over the window, a table with a mess of coffee cups and open biscuit packets and a small bookshelf. When he leaves the room to boil the kettle, I examine the books. They are all a call to arms, about every "ism" I've heard of – and some I haven't: capitalism, communism, socialism, fascism, feminism, unionism, authoritarianism, egalitarianism. I can't help asking about them and after each lesson we talk. Eventually, he lends me one, and we talk about it after the lesson. I'm enthralled. I failed to complete my journalism degree and have no real education beyond high school, where my focus was literature, not politics.

Like me, Rik comes from an immigrant family, and like me he felt responsible for his mother, who went mad with grief after the suicide of her middle son, eventually ending up in care, leaving the 14-year-old Rik to fend for himself, as by then his older brother had married. His father, a Communist sympathiser, had been forced to work in a German factory after the Nazi invasion of Holland during World War Two, as part of Arbeitseinsatz (Labour deployment) where he had died as the result of malnutrition and mistreatment. When his mother recovered, she returned to Holland. A year later, Rik joined her, studying guitar at a local conservatory. Before he finished the course, he was promoted to teacher in recognition of his talent. He returned to Melbourne at 24, with a young wife named Eva, whom he met in Belgium and who was keen to immigrate to Australia. But without a full qualification, he couldn't get a position teaching at university or at high school. He taught from home, reverting to the dole during the school holidays when there were no students. He and Eva had since divorced, but remained friends. He sometimes saw his older brother, who had a wife and two little boys, but he had no other family in Australia.

My family story feels tame beside his, but I tell him anyway. I also tell him why I wear long dresses.

"Don't you believe you're lovable?" Rik asks. Until then, I didn't.

"I think I'm falling for my guitar teacher," I tell my friend Sally, who like Jenny and John, is a volunteer at Learning Exchange.

The books Rik lends me, and our discussions, give me a language for my natural empathy for the underdog. We begin to spend more time talking than playing guitar, until one night we part with a kiss, instead of our usual goodbye.

"You're like me – intense," he says, gazing down at me.

With every lesson, things become more intense.

"Don't you believe you deserve to be happy?" Rik says when I tell him how I tried to leave Danny but couldn't.

A few weeks later, I arrive home in Bates Street at seven in the morning. Danny is sitting up in bed, looking stricken.

"Where have you been?" he asks, and I realise with a pang that he has worried all night.

"With Rik," I say, as I lay beside him, buzzing with spent passion.

"Do you love him?" he asks.

"Yes."

My separation from Danny a few months later doesn't surprise Mum.

"He had no ambition," she says.

14

The only things I take from my life with Danny are my books and clothes, my cane chair, my old pedal organ, the small framed picture of the *Le Musician* – the talisman for the life I craved and will now have with Rik – and a floral plate with a navy blue and gold border. Shirley carried that plate all the way from Pennsylvania as a gift for me when she visited her daughter in the US. I will miss her the most.

I'm sad and sorry, but I'm also in love. I'm going to have a new life with Rik – a man with a guitar and a bookshelf full of ideas, who was there for his mother when she suffered tragedy, just as I was there for mine. His mother's plight, his brother's death and his father's experience as a communist opened Rik's eyes to the problems of the ordinary working man and the need for social change, which feels like an extension of the feminism I always supported; liberation not just for women, but for everyone. Together we'll brave an unjust world.

Except, at the last minute, Rik changes his mind. It's too soon to move in together, he says. That wasn't his understanding. My heart sinks, but perhaps he's right. No need to rush things. I rent a one-bedroom flat in Jolimont, a short walk through the Fitzroy Gardens to my job at *The Herald*, and move in alone late one autumn afternoon.

It's Friday night and as I unpack my new doona to make up my new bed, I realise I've forgotten to buy sheets, so I walk back through the gardens to Myer in Swanston Street, which is open for late night shopping. The descending darkness has drained the colour from the trees. The city workers, bent forward in their haste to get home, look past me, focused on the next step that will take them to the station, the suburb, the person and the life waiting for them. No one is waiting for me as I walk back, past the possums brazenly raiding the overflowing bins.

I have no contact with family, except Mum and Walter, who are busy with their own life. Being married set me apart from my mostly single colleagues at *The Herald*. Being suddenly unmarried doesn't change their view or mine that we're on different paths. Jenny and John are torn between their loyalty to Danny and their loyalty to me and haven't warmed to Rik, or he to them. My friend Sally, whom I confided in, went around to comfort Danny and stayed.

"It's so weird to see Sally sitting on your couch with Danny," John says, the one time we catch up.

Just as I replace Danny, Danny replaces me. I'm not surprised. Sally was single for a long time. Danny is suddenly single and in shock. It's convenient. But the thought that I'm so replaceable makes me even more insecure. What did almost seven years of marriage mean to either of us? As I walk back with my purchase through the gardens in the dark, my heart begins to race, as if I'm being pursued. I'm not, of course. No one is pursuing me, not even Rik. I don't know this is a panic attack. All I know is I'm 26, suddenly single and "not coping", as Mum would say. Not coping is unacceptable. You have to "get on with it", so I trudge up the stairs to my new flat with my purchase, turn the key in the lock and walk into my new life with less confidence than I walked out of the old one.

"I'd forgotten what it's like to have clean sheets," Rik says when he visits the next night.

Clean sheets and home-cooked meals are not enough. When he told me to seize the happiness I deserved, he didn't mean it would be found with him. Rik always has his own plans, and mostly they don't include me. If he stays on Friday night, he leaves the next morning, explaining that he's going to a Dutch movie, or to his favourite Bulgarian restaurant, which serves his favourite Cevapi sausages.

"You can come along if you like," he sometimes says, when he sees my disappointed face. We take my car. He's swapped his for a 250cc motorbike, which is cheaper to run. But he never graduates beyond L Plates, so isn't permitted to carry a pillion passenger.

Gratefully, I tag along; driving the car but not the agenda, always on my best behaviour to ensure that lunch might extend to dinner and perhaps another overnight stay.

I want certainty. He wants freedom.

"What's the big fucking tragedy?" he asks in exasperation one night as I lay beside him on the mattress on the floor, my feelings of rejection erupting in quiet sobs. He often told me how his mother's tears were a game to manipulate him into pity, and he views mine the same way. His cool rationality paralyses me. Meeting Eva, his former wife, doesn't help. Warm and as wholesome as the bread she bakes, Eva is the living example of Rik's ability to move on.

"Would you like to see my house?" she says, as we sit sipping tea in her upstairs room in St Kilda, and she hands me a photo of herself – naked – hauling mudbricks with her friends for the house she's building at the Moora Moora Cooperative near Healesville. We don't have much in common apart from Rik, but I admire her ability to build her own house, even more so with no clothes on.

Unwittingly, I've repeated the very thing that dislocated me as a teenager when my mother severed all contact with the rest of our family. Without Danny's family, I feel the loss and absence of my own family for the first time. Work is my salvation, but there, too, I'm an observer, not a participator, reporting on the lives of others. My sense of loss is reflected in the stories I write. A story about the sculptor William Ricketts, old, frail and struggling to remain in his mountain retreat, is written with such empathy that one of the nameless sub editors who toils away behind the scenes suddenly appears at my desk with my story and a stunned look: "This is really good," he says.

Sometimes on lonely Sundays I call Mum, my voice low and flat, and confess I feel strange and sad.

"It'll pass," she says.

In her new home in Elwood with Walter, she's busy supervising a kitchen renovation, turning it from a bachelor's flat into something presentable enough to entertain their many friends. Once, when I'm riding the "down" escalator in Myer's, I'm surprised to see her gliding past on the "up" escalator. At least I think it's her. Her long straight black hair is clown-like: short, curly and ginger.

"Do you like it?" she asks when I wave her down and we meet on the ground floor.

"It's a wig."

She's thinking of getting a perm, and this is a test. A week or so later when we meet for coffee, her black hair forms a frizzy halo around her painted face. Walter obviously drew the line at ginger.

When Rik and Mum finally meet at afternoon tea with Walter at Milton Street, Mum is gracious and charming, which makes me nervous. I've seen her unmasking her guests at parties, while carefully maintaining her own, and I know what she's up to. Rik speaks fluent Dutch and German as well as fluent English; he reads the left-wing Dutch magazine *Vrij Nederland* in Dutch *Der Spiegel* magazine in German and Karl Marx in English. He also speaks another language with which she is familiar: music. I hope she'll be impressed. I watch anxiously as she teases out information about his work prospects (none), his family (almost none) and his ambitions (none). Danny – Mark 2. But not to me. To me, Rik is creative, interesting and non-conformist. With loads of potential.

The pattern of advance and retreat between Rik and me becomes normal, so I'm surprised when he suggests we rent a cabin at Wilson's Promontory one long weekend. I'm glad it's winter, not swimming weather. I look forward to cuddling up together in front of an open fire, talking books and movies. But Rik is strangely quiet.

"What's wrong?" I ask.

"I've got something to tell you," he says.

This is it. He's going to break up with me.

He takes a small silver sheet of small white tablets from his back pocket.

"I take these to help me relax."

The tablets are tranquilisers, a form of diazepam called Serapax. He's taking eight a day, but that weekend he hasn't taken any, as he's decided to give up.

Relief! I'm not the problem. Compassion! He's trying to be a better person. Joy! We have one more thing in common: anxiety.

As soon as we return home, he admits himself as a voluntary patient in a psychiatric hospital in Parkville. But he hates the locked doors and punitive atmosphere and leaves three days later. He'll go it alone. Except that doesn't work either, and soon he returns to the Rik I know and love – intelligent, sensitive, rational, idealistic and emotionally unavailable.

Loneliness and compassion keep me there. Rik is a man with a guitar, with a European background and a fraught family: intriguingly different – and familiar. Just like Danny, he listens to 3CR, but instead of *Nostalgia Unlimited* every Saturday morning we listen to a Dario Fo play every Saturday morning called, *We Can't Pay, We Won't Pay*, where housewives revolt against the rising prices at a supermarket. Rik confesses he's been revolting for a while. When he and Eva were short of cash in their marriage, he sometimes wore his special long coat with the holes in the pockets to his own local supermarket, where small items fell conveniently into the hem, undetected. Once he had the nerve to return a rancid camembert and demand a refund. I know it's wrong, but I can't help admiring his audacity and ingenuity, in the same way I'd secretly admired my father's. The fruits of capitalism should be shared by all. Couched in the terms of worker versus the capitalist, it feels just.

Like the protagonists in the play, Rik isn't just questioning the system; he and his friend Harry Van Moorst, a Footscray academic, plan to change it. Harry founded The Coalition against Poverty and Unemployment, which is frequently quoted in the media as an authority on the problems of the poor.

Although I often write about the poor in the sob stories for *The Herald*, I'm woefully ignorant about how they got that way. *The Herald* and its sister paper *The Sun* are big on promoting the causes of Little Aussie Battlers, but neither ever suggests any real change to reduce the number of battles they face. Sometimes, they even make them worse. Once, as a general reporter, I wrote a story about a mother of a disabled child who claimed the Royal Children's Hospital denied her child treatment at birth. But the story was tweaked to imply the hospital had saved the child's life. When *The Herald* used the story to promote the hospital's Good Friday Appeal, I declined a byline and left the office for the day, walking around the city in furious tears.

Yet I have no real understanding of the forces behind such decisions. Nor do I question, as Rik does, why people have to stand on the street shaking tins to raise money for an essential service like the Children's Hospital.

"You're uninformed," Rik tells me.

He's right. My new position as local government reporter puts many of my stories on the front page, but I'm ignorant about party politics. When *The Herald* asks me to write an opinion piece commenting on the Melbourne City Council elections, I ring my trusty contact, a wily former Labor Lord Mayor from the former sacked council. It's no surprise to anyone except me when he and most of the former Labor council are re-elected.

But it's the "union bashing," that upsets Rik.

"*The Herald* is a right-wing rag," he says. I begin to be ashamed of the stories I was once proud of. My boss and colleagues at *The Herald* blink in amazement when six months later I hand in my resignation and accept a new job at a new local paper – *The Western Times*, started by a journalist friend and her husband. I will return to cartooning – and practise a more respectable form of journalism in a Labor heartland.

Unlike the Sandringham paper I'd edited for Standard News, where I had to coax stories out of the well-to-do residents who had the money to solve their problems privately, in the west the poor were in the streets and at the office door, clamouring for publicity about the lack of housing, roads, education, and employment – and the proliferation consumer rip offs.

With the help of Carolyn Bond, a local financial counsellor who provides the case studies, I start a column called Consumer Casebook, giving voice to all the people who've been ripped off by the system.

"We don't need the story now. The cartoon says it all," the sub-editor at *The Times* says after I submit a cartoon – for my story about a dodgy weight-loss company – of a fat woman with her purse, followed by a cartoon of the same fat woman without her purse.

Changing the world is easy. Changing myself isn't.

"How come you're still wearing long dresses?" Rik asks one day.

"What's the big deal?"

"People stare."

"That's their problem," he says

Later that week, I stand in front of the long mirror at home and lift my skirt, contemplating Rik's suggestion for a trial run – wearing a short dress for a few hours the following Friday night. In the dark, my right leg might look the same as my left – to anyone who's had a few drinks – or something stronger.

The next night, Rik takes out the little foil blister packet of Serapax from his back pocket and removes one tablet, breaking it in half. I swallow it and change into the soft grey knee-length cotton check dress bought for $20 at the market, along with a pair of sheer panty hose to cover my brown compression stocking.

"Where are we going?" I smile half an hour later as I sit in the car feeling naked and exposed.

"To Eva's."

Of course, Eva – the perfect role model for not caring about being naked.

While Eva serves us tea, Rik gives me the second half of the tablet. An hour later I follow him outside to Chapel Street. The warm night air licks deliciously around my stockinged legs. I stare defensively ahead, clutching Rik's arm, daring the oncoming crowds of shoppers to stare back.

Nobody does. I'm naked and nobody notices. So, this is what it's like to feel normal? Almost.

"When will the bandages be removed from your ankle?" a friend asks a few weeks later. I sit wearing my short grey dress, with my legs elegantly crossed as we chat over a glass of wine. "There are no bandages," I explain. "That's my ankle."

I don't blame her. Nor do I blame the old man at the market who exclaims loudly, "Mamma mia! What's a-wrong with ya foots?"

I continue to wear short dresses; it's so much easier. I no longer have to make my own clothes. I simply avoid situations where the opportunity to comment is greatest, such as Japanese restaurants where you have to remove your shoes and line them up at the entrance for all to see, or at events with children, who have no filters and always gawp, or ask questions, such as "Why is your foot fat?"

Nothing's really changed, except it no longer matters. I'm normal enough. And because I never mention it, my work colleagues and the people I interview don't either. I'm more interested in my work. The Consumer Casebook I create with Carolyn gives me a swag of good stories and contacts with people I admire, who are activists in practice, not just theory.

"See ya," Carolyn says one day after work as we cross the road outside the office together. As she turns away, I have a sudden regret that she regards me as a colleague rather than a friend. The women in CAPU are part of my friendship group, but our contact is mostly limited to political meetings. We don't hang out together. Nor am I part of the sisterhood, the feminist movement of the time. I have no real sister either – at least not that I see – and since Jenny and John have gone to Europe for a year to fulfil their dream, and there are no other female reporters at *The Western Times*, I have no real girlfriends I can make sisters of.

"Hey," I call out as Carolyn begins to disappear into the crowd. "Do you want to go out for lunch or a coffee some time?"

"That'd be nice," she calls back. My heart soars. We begin to meet regularly, exchanging stories about our lives and families, as well as her clients for Consumer Casebook. Carolyn has a sister, whom she sees regularly. I tell her about the one I don't see, and as always, I make a dinner-party joke of our family estrangement, and don't speak of it again.

Three months later, Carolyn invites me to join her on a trip to Europe, starting with England first, where she has relatives. Whenever anyone asks if I'm Italian, I feel like an imposter. I look Italian, I have the nose and the name, but I don't speak it and have never been there. This is my chance. I will go to England with Carolyn and on to Italy to find out if I'm a "real Cafarella". I half hope Rik will come too, and we can tour Holland together, but he has no money and never asks, so I don't invite him.

Four weeks before the trip, on a cold winter's night in June, Rik and I are celebrating his birthday on the mattress on the floor in the room he rents in his shared house when the condom breaks.

"It'll probably be a little Jane," he jokes.

Six weeks later the joke is on me. I feel a pang of regret when Rik says he doesn't want a little Jane or a little Rik, and we agree on an abortion. I'm used to assuming it's impossible for me to have a child. Besides, I have my pack and my passport for my trip with Carolyn. I don't confide in her about it. I will deal with it as I have before, privately, before the trip.

Strangely, this decision doesn't give me the same sense of liberation I had in the same situation with Danny. I'm weighed down with inexplicable unbearable regret. My sister Julie has a baby, although I know nothing about her experiences of motherhood. Gail has one, too. In the year before I left Danny, she married her former

Hari Krishna boyfriend and gave birth to a boy with golden curls, the image of his father. I've seen photos of Rik as a sweet earnest child, and my heart secretly yearns for a little Rik, though I don't admit it.

In my heart I know he's right. He has casual employment, a tranquilliser addiction and smokes a packet of cigarettes a day. He isn't fully committed to me. How will he cope with a child? But every time we sit down to eat, I choke on my unspoken words, and the tension between us follows us like a cloud as we drift between our two shared houses.

A week before my appointment, we go away for the weekend to Craig's Hotel, in Ballarat, to clear the air. The bridal suite is the only room available. Most of the rooms are rented by a bunch of drunken Rotarians, who spend the night whooping and yelling in the corridors. The air is heavy with Rik's repressed anger and my repressed longing as we sit on the edge of grand four-poster bed together. It's now or never.

"I've got something to tell you," I say, my heart hammering.

"What?"

"I've changed my mind."

The cloud hanging over us becomes thunderous.

"You can't just decide this," Rik says. "You just can't make a decision that affects my life without consulting me."

I breathlessly explain what's possible, while he explains with glacial rationality what's impossible.

"We'd made an agreement," he says. "You've got no right to break it."

We drive home in pitiless silence, every kilometre bringing me closer to the appointment and the place I so blithely went to get rid of the babies I hadn't wanted with Danny.

Two days before the appointed day, I'm sitting in the kitchen at Rik's place with his housemate Sue, as she chatters on while energetically packing vegetables into Tupperware containers to transfer to the fridge. I can barely raise a smile, and though I try to hide it with cold-water splashes, my face is bloated from crying.

Sue stops suddenly, mid Tupperware, and examines me with sudden interest. "You're not pregnant, are you?"

"Yes," I sob. She makes me a cup of tea, which I dilute with my tears as I tell her the whole story.

"You need to get some advice," she says, and she hands me the address of an organisation I've never heard of – The Council for the Single Mother and her Child. "They help single mothers."

Single mothers! I'm not going to be a single mother. I'm happy to write about them sympathetically, but I don't want to be one. Sue smiles and tells me to go anyway.

The Council for the Single Mother and Her Child is in a big room upstairs in Flinders Lane, cosy with books, magazines and children's toys and comfy old couches facing each other over an old wooden coffee table. Two women, not much older than me, make me coffee and stare incredulously as I explain how I can't have this baby because the father won't agree.

"But you've got a good job," they say. "So what if he doesn't want it? So what if you've got a ticket to go around the world? Take your baby with you."

It's as if I've been standing outside a door that has suddenly been flung open. I do have a good job, which gives me choices I haven't realised. Everything seems possible – except telling Rik. I tell my boss's wife instead. "God will provide," she says solemnly. I don't believe in God. Not since childhood, when my father exclaimed, "May God strike me dead," when he lied to my mother, about which God did absolutely nothing. I know I'll be the one providing, but that's okay. I have a good job, a car and a round-the world ticket to freedom.

I cancel the abortion. I'm relieved, terrified and suddenly fearless. This is no longer just about me. It's two against one. I ring Rik and tell him matter-of-factly I'm going ahead with this pregnancy and while I'll keep him informed of the child's progress, I don't require his involvement.

He seems surprised. I'm surprised, too, and a little sad and scared when he agrees. Carolyn goes to London without me and I haunt the baby department at Myer searching for clues about the new life I've chosen. I try to imagine who this child will be, and who I'll be when I become a mother. Regardless of Rik's failure to commit, I hope this child will be just like its father: musical, with two perfect legs.

Telling Rik is hard enough. Now I have to tell Mum. She's still living with Walter in Elwood, working part-time at the tennis centre at Malvern, where she takes Possum, the baby that will never grow up. I know she won't approve. A single mother! My courage begins to feel foolish, even irresponsible. How can I work and pay for a child? Will the newly legislated single mother's pension cover the rent? What if I'm evicted? I know from the reception I'd received from Mum when I landed on her doorstep when I tried to leave Danny that I'd find no refuge with her. And what about Walter? He's a rather stiff and formal man who never says anything other than "I'll get Mum," followed by his customary nervous laugh when I telephone each week.

Before I have a chance to call her, Rik calls me.

"I can't let you do this alone. You'll probably fuck it up," he says.

15

Rik stares at the list I've written of people to call about the happy news.

"Why do we have to let them know? Won't they just see the baby when we're out walking with the pram?" he says, frowning.

"It's tradition," I say. Why doesn't he understand that friends and family expect to be informed that we are now the proud parents of a "little Rik", with two perfect legs? Except not my father or sister. They aren't on the list or my mind. They exist in the past, not the present. I visited my sister at the birth of her daughter, but I don't expect her to visit me at the birth of my son. Since Nanny's death, the connection between "Camp Doris and Dad" and my world has broken. The present is full of new family and new friends, who, like me, are in love with this "infant joy".

Together Rik and I chose a pine cot and a cherry red pram, swapping trepidation and resistance for acceptance and excitement in the semi-detached three-bedroom house we rent in Bellair Street, Kensington.

"You don't know how lucky you are to have a healthy baby," Mum says, when she visits me in hospital a few days after the birth. Every mother is luckier than her, with her two sick babies poisoned by her monkey blood.

"Where's Rik working?" she asks, feigning nonchalance.

"Still teaching," I say, although this is only half true. He is suffering from Carpel Tunnel Syndrome and no amount of plunging his wrists into icy water alleviates the pain. I've left the *Western Times* for a short-term job at Consumer Affairs, which conveniently ended in time for the birth. We're living on my savings and whatever he can earn when he's able. I'm not worried about money. I can go back to journalism any time. Babies don't need much, especially the son of humble workers like us, happy to eschew the ill-gotten gains of capitalism.

"It'll be okay," I say,

Mum raises a drawn-on eyebrow as she regards her grandson.

"You'll want to do things for him and buy things for him."

I don't reply. She greeted the news of my pregnancy with the same guarded neutrality that she had greeted my marriage to Danny and my decision to leave him for Rik. Just as we didn't do wedding things together, we didn't do baby things together. The only interest she showed was in his name – Jakob, pronounced with a Y – a beautiful Dutch name to go with Rik's Dutch surname.

"I'll call him 'Jacky'," she said when I told her.

"No, you won't," I said, my face flushing at such desecration.

"Yes, I will."

"You won't."

Silence.

"What will I call him then?"

"By his name."

And she does. Although she never can pronounce it properly.

Back in our little house in Bellair Street in Kensington, Rik and I take turns to pace the hall on colicky nights while playing Bach cello suites to sooth our son to sleep. Eva knits baby clothes for him, my friend Jenny crochets a cot blanket for him from wool she grows and spins herself, and Rik goes off Serapax for him – cold turkey. I buy Rik *Winnie the Pooh*, to help him reclaim his own lost childhood and he buys me short stories by Franz Kafka. Together we read *The Metamorphosis*, to further educate me.

Lying on the loungeroom floor with Jakob splayed on my breast, I am as content, fecund and bountiful as a cow. Motherhood isn't a trap after all. It's a door to a new sparkling world of true love and discovery.

"When do you put him down?" the maternal and child health nurse asks during a routine visit.

Put him down? I don't put him down. When Rik gets a job at the Tenant's Union in Footscray, helping the poor, I dress Jakob up and go out for the day – to parks, gardens, lullaby workshops and shows, discovering the world anew – and that it's truly a man's world. The broken footpaths in Kensington make walking with the cherry-red pram a roller coaster ride. There are no baby seats on shopping trolleys and the local supermarket doesn't allow prams in the aisles. The pram is too wide for the narrow doorway at the local post office and it's impossible to go to a public toilet unless some kind stranger (who you hope isn't also a kidnapper) agrees to wait outside the cubicle and guard the pram. It's as if I've woken up on a different planet, where it's women and children last. Doesn't the world realise that the sun rises every day in our house alone, and it needs to adjust itself?

Neither the world nor my mother adjusts.

"What are you doing here?" she asks in alarm, when I drop in on the way back from the city one dinnertime, my breasts bursting and the baby screaming. I feed him hastily and leave, feeling like an intruder.

"He weed on my shirt," she says, the first and only time I ask her to look after him. "We couldn't go out anywhere because I couldn't open the pusher. It was impossible!"

I don't ask again. Instead, I ring each week to gush over his progress.

"It's a pity I can't see him," she says.

"Why not?"

"You're so far away."

Far away? I'm in Kensington. She's in Elwood – a 30-minute drive away.

"Such a pity," she says, and even though I look up train and tram routes for her, our weekly phone calls remain our main contact.

Part of me feels I deserve her disinterest. Although she doesn't say it, I know by her pursed lips and inquisitorial eyebrow that she feels I've made bad choices, marrying too young, having abortions, divorcing Danny and having a child out of wedlock – all by the age of 27, although having a child out of wedlock doesn't bother me except that it may bother her. She remains a visitor, and once again I attach myself to a new family – spending weekends visiting Rik's brother and his partner, who share our political views, and who have two little boys of their own.

Early one Sunday morning, as Rik and I are finishing breakfast, the phone rings.

"It's Dad," the voice says. "Nonna died."

"I'm sorry," I say, my heart thudding, as I tried to register a death and a resurrection in one phone call.

My Aunt Tess gave him my number, he explains.

I never knew Dad's mother as "Nonna". To my sister Julie and me she was Nana Cafarella, who with her warm brown eyes and short cropped white hair, sat fanning herself at Aunty Mary's, calling us her "chickens", in a throaty chuckle exacerbated by asthma, and for whom Dad bought a bedraggled bunch of chrysanthemums from a roadside trader every Mother's Day.

"You like, I make!" Nana says when I am 14 and I admire the delicate biscuit-coloured doilies she crochets. I like so much that she offers to teach me, although Mum is unimpressed. "Why do you want to learn that?" she says.

Years earlier, as a new journalist, I learned the surprising facts of Nana's life when I interviewed her in her flat in Essendon – how she had been raised by a wicked stepmother on the island of Salina in Sicily after a jealous woman had cursed her lovely young mother with "malocchio" – the evil eye. Lured by tales of "terra dora" (streets of gold), she came to Australia in 1923 with her father in the first Italian diaspora.

"What did you think when you got here? I'd asked.

"You know, I was so disappoint," she said.

Yet, as my father explains the funeral arrangements, there is another pull – of loyalty to my mother, betrayed by her own family and forgotten by my father's. I hope Nana Cafarella is in the heaven in which she so fervently believed, with her beloved saints, as I explain I won't be attending her funeral. I have to work.

My father suggests we meet the following week instead.

"It'll be good to see you," he says.

* * *

I recognise him at once, sitting in the back at Genevieve's Café in Carlton, expertly lighting a cigarette with the pincer thumb of his fingerless left hand.

He doesn't recognise me.

"Have you got false teeth?" he asks, as I sit down, nervously clutching my handbag with the photo of my 12-month-old son I bring to show him.

"No," I say suddenly self-conscious. They're the same teeth I've always had.

He's full of news about the big house with the sweeping beach views he's building with his one-and-half hands for Doris in Fairhaven, to replace the house that was razed in the Ash Wednesday bushfires three years earlier.

"It's been bloody awful, what with the insurance claims and all," he says, tapping his cigarette on the ashtray.

He pauses and says matter-of-factly. "Doris discovered condoms in my briefcase."

Condoms? I stare at him in puzzled disbelief. Of all the things my mother accused him of when I was growing up, infidelity seemed the least probable. He always seemed more interested in cars than women.

"It's all fine now," he says, lighting another cigarette, and he tells me about the newsagency they've bought in Geelong and of their life together.

I leave with the photo of my son still in my bag, the stench of cigarettes and disappointment in my clothes.

Shortly after, as I'm trying to catch some sleep before picking Jakob up from creche, there's another phone call. "There's been an accident."

Someone left a narrow unframed mirror leaning against a sofa at the crèche and it fell on Jakob, slicing his top lip open.

"Just as well he's a boy and can grow a moustache to cover the scar," the doctor at the Royal Children's Hospital says after stitching the wound. Jakob is fine, but I'm not. I can't stop crying. Beauty and innocence have been patched but not restored. I want to sue the crèche. The more I cry, the angrier Rik becomes.

"You're being fucking bitchy," he says.

I am puzzled and hurt that he isn't on my side – our side.

Distraught, I apply for a week's leave from my new job working on projects for Children's Week at the Premier's Department, explaining that I need to care for our son when he's discharged from hospital.

"Even if he'd died, you're only entitled to three days leave," my manager says. Outraged, I take permanent leave and the first job I can find – as a part-time reporter at *The Sunday Press* – another "right-wing rag" in Rik's view. My left-wing friends are delighted. I've infiltrated a capitalist enclave. But I'm embarrassed when my sympathetic stories about struggling sole parents and tenants are given snide subheadings such as "Your taxes at work".

When a colleague mentions *The Age* is looking for sub-editors and to call someone called "Millo" after six pm, I jump. It's night shift and will fit in well with caring for my son during the day. It's also prestigious. *The Age* practises the sort of journalism I can be proud of.

"Cafarella! Lovely family!" "Millo" says when I call. "Come in!"

"Millo" is Bob Millington, a popular *Age* columnist and the chief night sub-editor. He knows my Aunt Tess, who taught his brother. It's the first time the name Cafarella has ever opened a door for me.

* * *

I am a terrible sub. I'm hired on the strength of my *Herald* stories, not my subbing skills. "If I've told you once, I've told you a hundred times," the "check" sub yells night after night, thumping his fist on the desk, when I continue to flout the rules about "Americanisms" or make style errors. I've had no formal training. Nor have I ever used any computer system. I'm flying by the seat of my pants. Every morning after my shift I snatch four hours' sleep and get up with an energetic toddler. I have no time to fully inform myself of the day's events for the stories I am subbing that night, despite the help of Lisa, a kindly Chilean woman in her 50s, who comes once a week to help with housework.

After about six months, the deputy chief sub takes me aside. "You've got to stop talking about your son," he says.

"What?"

I'm talking too much and about the wrong thing, and it's affecting my work, which is not up to scratch, he says.

I am mortified, but I understand. I'm a fraud. What I don't understand is how this warning has been framed, and why it's okay for the male subs to bore me stupid with their talk of golf, but not okay for me to bore them equally stupid with my tales of motherhood.

The rage I felt at discovering the incompatibility of the physical world with motherhood is ignited by this new injustice. Furious, I pound out a passionate story pointing out that, despite the gains of women's liberation, the world still refuses to recognise and accommodate the real needs of mothers and children – and submit it to Accent, *The Age's* women's section.

"A mother's fighting words" the headline cries. I keep my job as a sub, and accept the invitation from the Accent editor to write freelance stories for the section.

I have no such fighting words at home.

"Can I borrow some of your records?" Rik asks as we eat dinner one night.

"Yes, why?"

I'm flattered. Rik's taste in music has always seemed so much more sophisticated than mine.

"I'm going around to Maria's," he says.

Maria is a work colleague, he explains. He's going around to play my records – and stay the night.

Stay the night? What does it mean?

"Why does it have to mean anything?" he says.

It may mean he no longer loves me. It may mean he's going to leave me for this person, I reply.

He regards me with bemusement. "You're telling me I can only love one person?"

I'm telling him I'm confused, hurt, and threatened, but in the face of his claims that I'm putting a limit on love I have no argument.

"You're being controlling," he says, and he takes my records and leaves.

I rationalise that he's going through an identity crisis, as he can no longer play guitar. I rationalise it's my fault. I am controlling. Didn't I object when he lay on the bed as soon as I made it? I am a perfectionist, except when it comes to my appearance. A failed perm has made my fine hair short and frizzy. I've put on weight – as Rik notes. Grey circles underline my eyes, which I can hardly keep open, thanks to the double shift of early mornings and late nights. A few weeks later, as we prepare to go shopping, Rik points to my three-quarter length yellow cotton elastic-waisted pants.

"What's with the fucking half-mast pants?"

Like most of the three-quarter pants in fashion, they expose my big foot. I am stung. Since "coming out" and wearing short dresses, I've convinced myself no one notices.

"I love you despite your leg. Not because of it," Rik explains.

I don't object. We have other things to argue about – like money. He wants to buy a vibraphone. We can't afford it and I can't see how hitting keys with a rubber mallet will be any easier on his painful wrists than playing guitar. We're at an impasse. Like all such arguments, it's a symptom rather than the cause of our disintegrating relationship. I should leave. He should leave. But we have a child together, so we endure, our unspent rage and frustration simmering but never quite boiling over – until one Sunday afternoon.

We argue again. Rik is lying on the couch with his eyes closed. Calm. Impassive. Rational. The colour television we couldn't afford mutters away in the background. I take his glass of beer from the nearby table and pour it over his face.

***

"Come, come!" Lisa says when she opens the door of her Housing Commission flat and sees me standing with Jakob in my arms, my face swollen and bruised.

Lisa and I have never shared more than a few polite words during her weekly visit to help with the housework, but something in her face as we'd worked together had told me she'd known trouble.

In broken English she explains she's never been happier since she left her abusive husband. I'm shocked. Rik isn't an abusive husband. This has never happened before. It probably wouldn't have happened at all if I hadn't provoked him by pouring the beer over his face. I'm sure it'll never happen again. He's a loving father to our son, even if our relationship is tense. Lisa shakes her head and sighs.

It never occurs to me to seek help from my mother. The previous year she and Walter had married in a small ceremony at The Mint in Melbourne, attended by my stepsisters, Amanda and Jeanette, and me.

"Do you think I should do it?" she asked the week before the wedding.

"You've been together nine years. What's the difference?" I said.

In the photo they give us afterwards, she is seated in the garden, wearing a silvery-grey satin blouse, raising her long hot pink satin skirt coquettishly to reveal a cheeky frilly pink garter. She is 59.

Marriage is both a stress and a relief. "I've come to this marriage with nothing," she laments whenever I call, and to prove her worth she becomes an exemplary wife and a charming hostess, always beautifully dressed and coiffed, turning out cuisine extraordinaire for Walter and their friends, despite a tight budget.

I'm too ashamed to go to my friend Carolyn's. I know Carolyn considers Rik a loser and will urge me to leave. I thank Lisa as she makes up a bed for me and Jakob on a beanbag in the corner of the lounge room, where he sleeps and I lie awake.

16

The plastic bucket full of sodden nappies cuts into my fingers as I trudge over the sandy hillocks to the amenities block in Apollo Bay, along the rugged coastline of the Great Ocean Road. In the distance, a man in a wetsuit, a gleaming white surfboard tucked neatly under his arm, ambles across the sand. I watch as he wades into the waiting waves, lies on the board and paddles out to sea before attempting a wobbly stand.

I'd already fought against a vibraphone, with drastic results. Who was I to argue about a surfboard?

Rik and I are on a healing holiday at Apollo Bay on the Great Ocean Road. As Plato said: "The sea cures all the ailments of man."

It's three months since I sought refuge with Lisa. I had returned to Bellair Street the following morning, and our life together resumed under a cloud of humiliation and unspoken shame. The domestic violence I so often wrote about is now real to me, along with the reasons women who should leave don't. Unlike many of the women I write about, I have the means to leave, but like generations of women before me, I'm determined to keep my family together – at any cost.

I wring out the clean nappies and hang them to dry in the sea air.

A few days later, Rik turns to me as we sit up in bed in our seaside apartment, with Jakob jumping excitedly between us.

"I wanna split," Rik says.

I stare at him. "Split, as in go home?"

"Split, as in split up," he says.

I stare in disbelief. It isn't personal, he says. He just needs to do his own thing, to be creative. Alone.

"Alone? But we're a family."

"We'll still be a family," he says. "I'll have Jakob half the week and you can have him the other half."

He has it all worked out, this half-life for us all, even what we'll tell the rest of the family and friends: that it's amicable, mature and for the best – for our son's sake. The healing sea, symbol of changing moods, has turned and I am drowning. In the remaining days of our holiday, I cling to Rik like a barnacle on a boat.

"You're feeling sad, aren't you?" he observes, with no hint of sadness himself, as we lie in bed together. To oblige me, we make love. I feel ashamed and grateful as I give myself up to grief and to pretending he still wants me.

Six weeks later, I juggle Jakob on my knee, as the local doctor tells me what I don't want to believe. I am pregnant – and alone. Rik has moved out. Our house in Bellair Street is a mess of boxes and newspaper as I pack to move with Jakob across the railway line to a two-bedroom flat I've rented in Eastwood Street.

"The agreement was that we share the parenting of one child, not two," Rik says sternly and rationally when I tell him about the pregnancy. It's not negotiable. If I go ahead, he will deny paternity.

It's Solomon's choice.

I weep as I recall my mother's words: "There's a price for everything."

Jakob and I stay in the flat in Eastwood Street and Rik rents a flat in Brunswick Road, where he stores the forgotten surfboard in the pantry and we fall into a pattern of shared care.

Soon after the crèche rings to tell me Jakob has lice. That night, he refuses to let me wash the lice shampoo out of his hair, no matter how many jellybeans I give him. Furious, I drag him from the bath and dump him on his bed, and with all the pent-up rage I should have spent on Rik, I hit him.

The purple jellybean he's been chewing is suddenly visible on his purple tongue as he screams. I hit him again and, seeing his terror, I fall on him crying, pleading for forgiveness.

"I never liked him," my mother says, when I tell her that Rik and I are separating. I never tell her the real reasons.

* * *

The landlord, a short balding man in his 60s, is bent over the bath, fixing the tap.

"You can buy! Yes, you can. Ask your momma and poppa for $10,000," he says as he casually explains our flat in Eastwood Street is for sale. My son and I are about to be evicted.

The total asking price is $80,000 – a bargain for the near-new stylish two-bedroom flat in the heart of Kensington, the smiling landlord says.

I don't know whether to laugh or cry. I have a good job as a bad sub-editor at *The Age*, and some money saved, but nowhere near the $10,000 required for a deposit. I haven't seen or heard from my father since we met in the café two years earlier. I can't and won't ask him for money. I doubt he has any. I can't ask Mum either, who regularly reminds me how she came to her marriage with Walter with nothing. Walter owed his education to a scholarship at the prestigious Scotch College, where he excelled in "civics", maths and "penmanship" – an honour about which he regularly reminds everyone. His first wife was awarded the family home, and he's still working part-time to shore up income for retirement.

I have to find another flat to rent, despite the seed of desire for a place of my own that the landlord's suggestion has planted.

I'm late for my shift on the sub's desk. I decide to search for a new place tomorrow. I just have to get through this night, but with the word "eviction" racing around my head, I fear I'll be an even worse sub than usual.

I wait until the first edition has been "put to bed" at 11pm, when we all retreat to the "bog bar" in the men's locker room for a wine or a beer, before telling a colleague what the landlord had said.

"Why don't you?" she says.

"What?"

"Ask your parents."

She draws on her fag and sips her wine and looks at me quizzically. I sip my wine and stare back.

"Why not?" she insists. "You've got nothing to lose."

Why not, indeed? Fortified by wine and desperation, I pick up the phone. Mum answers: "Hello?"

I quickly explain that I know it's late, and everything's all right – well almost everything.

"Can you lend me $10,000 to buy the flat? I'm being evicted," I say, in a tone that suggests I don't really mean it.

Silence. I wait, my heart racing.

"Hang on. I'll ask Walter," she says. And she hangs up.

**

Mum is tight-lipped as she sweeps the small rectangle of lino in the kitchen of my new flat, bought with the money Walter lends me.

"You're not coping, are you?" she says.

She's right – and wrong. At work, I'm now a full-time reporter for Accent, the women's pages published on Wednesdays and Fridays in *The Age*, championing women from all walks of life. At home, I'm a lonely single mother with one failed relationship and two failed marriages behind me.

Yes. Two. One with Danny, and one on the rebound a year after Rik and I separate. This time, it's a man with a piano, not a guitar.

"Where have you been?" my new love panted after our first kiss. Where had I been? Through hell. Soon I was in heaven, courted with rippling arpeggios and romantic little notes written on restaurant napkins. It was clear that we should spend the rest of our lives together. We married on Valentine's Day at San Francisco City Hall where he was on business trip – and divorced a year later.

Together with my son, I move into the flat I buy in Flemington with the money Walter – the kindest man I've ever known – lends me. Our new flat, where Mum is sweeping my crunchy floor, is in a plain brown brick block with the ambitious name of Paris Court. In the loungeroom, Walter is pouring over Body Corporate documents to prevent another eviction – of the Burmese kitten I bought Jakob as a house-warming present, without realising that home-ownership didn't extend to cat ownership.

Despite Walter's efforts, our cat is evicted, but Jakob and I still have each other. On the weekends when it's my turn to have him, we curl up together watching musicals and eating lollies. On the weekends when he's with Rik, I haul potting mix and plants up the concrete stairs to the sunny north-facing balcony and create a garden of impatiens, climbing beans, tomatoes, a big pot containing two gold fish, and another sprouting a lonely corncob.

The balcony is my solace. The letterbox is my stress. Interest rates have climbed to 17-and-a-half per cent and every few weeks the bank sends another letter announcing another rise. There is no way I can begin to pay off Walter's loan. The previous Saturday while Jakob leaned on our shopping trolley at the market, I handed over my last 20 dollar note to pay for two kilos of potatoes – and received change of five.

I stared at the coins in my hand. "I gave you twenty," I said to the woman behind the stall.

"You gave me five," she said.

"That was supposed to pay for food for the week," I said, and I burst into tears.

The woman shrugged and handed me the rest of my change.

"Thank you," I spluttered, and went to buy a consoling donut to share with my son.

Such is the irrationality of having too many bills and too few comforts.

For further consolation, I take to my guitar.

"Don't you know any happy songs?" Jakob sobs in the bath as I sit on a stool beside him serenading him with *Black Girl* – a song about an abandoned girl in the pines where the sun never shines and who finds her father's severed head on the steering wheel.

Happy songs? I'm done with love and happy relationships. Outside home, my most rewarding relationship is with my readers. Every week for Accent, I interview women in politics, the arts, business, welfare and women making waves all over the world. When the copy falls short, I fill the gaps with quick cartoons, signing myself CAF, as Cafarella is too long.

Accent is popular with readers, but not with management, which regards it as an unnecessary aggravation. To protect it, the editor Rosemary West comes up with a brilliant plan – inviting readers to lunch at fancy hotels to hear prominent local and international speakers on issues important to women.

The first Accent lunch I attend is a celebration of International Women's Day featuring ABC presenter and former Accent reporter Ramona Koval, former president for the Movement for the Ordination of Women, Patricia Brennan, Director of the Koori Women's Centre at Monash University, Dr Eve Fesl, the first woman to be elected as a full-time industrial officer with the Trades Hall Council, Patricia Caswell, a lecturer in Women's Studies at the Deakin University Dr Robyn Rowland, comedian Mandy Solomon, my old friend Ian Macphee, the former first Minister for the Status of Women in the Fraser Government – and me, introducing them all.

That morning, my car breaks down. I walk my son to school and catch a taxi to the hotel, arriving just in time. Like the women speaking that day and the women I interview every day, I'm not about to give up.

But the stress of the previous few years comes out in other ways.

"It's the chair," I tell the night nurse at *The Age*, as she massages the painful knotty muscles in my back.

Despite my success at work, in my personal life I feel like a fool, lurching from one ill-thought-out relationship to the next. In a quiet moment at work, I dash off a cartoon in blue biro on a slip of copy paper, showing a woman putting out the garbage. On the two garbage bags are the words "My Life".

I'm surprised and flattered when *The Age* cartoonist Michael Leunig squats by my desk one day and invites me to submit a few cartoons for an exhibition at the Westpac Gallery at the Melbourne Arts Centre. I submit a cartoon about the advent of the "sensitive new man", with the caption "Sensitive to dust, sensitive to noise, and especially sensitive to criticism", and redraw the *My Life* cartoon with my favourite Artline 70 black pen.

I'm even more surprised to see *My Life* featured on the media release for the exhibition, which is titled, Cartoonists for Amnesty – along with a cartoon by popular *Age* cartoonist Ron Tandberg, whom I'd so brazenly imitated while trying to develop a style of my own.

When I attend the official opening, both my entries have red dots on them.

"Who bought them?" I ask, incredulous.

The curator smiles. "The State Library of Victoria."

A month later I'm asked to exhibit with a group of other cartoonists at the Roar2 Studios in Brunswick Street, Fitzroy.

My life is no longer rubbish.

17

Cartoons become my new freelance business, though most of the business comes from decidedly unfunny organisations – like the legal service where my friend Carolyn's husband Denis works, and mostly because I draw from a lefty feminist perspective and can churn them out by the dozen.

"Can I have a look?" the new young lawyer asks after following me into the photocopy room when I turn up to photocopy the cartoons Denis has commissioned.

"No," I say. I know my artistic limitations and am not sure he'll get the jokes.

"You can make me a cup of coffee." And he does.

"Hello, my name's Rob," he says, holding out his hand, while I sip my coffee.

I'm amused. Shaking hands seems like such an old-fashioned thing to do. I take a closer look: a bow tie with braces, blue-grey eyes behind glasses, brown curly corrugated hair, a putty nose, a deeply furrowed brow and open cheerful expression as if to say, "Here I am, ready to accept whoever you are."

I'm 33, pessimistic and cynical: a single mother with a five-year-old son, a broken heart and a history of serial marriage. I can barely accept myself, let alone anyone else.

"Nice to meet you," I say, shaking his hand, and I leave with my cartoons.

"Rob plays guitar," my friend Carolyn says the next week as we share a glass of wine at her place in Essendon. I prick up my ears, and then check myself. Another man with a guitar. Never!

A few weeks later, I'm invited to a party. "Rob will be there," Carolyn says.

I'm not a party girl, but Rik has Jakob that weekend and I don't want to spend it in the flat on my own. Rob isn't at the party, but another young lawyer with a guitar is. His name is Bevan, and he knows all the old Joan Baez songs my parents sang, so, naturally, I invite him over for a Sunday jam.

"Do you mind if I bring a friend?" Bevan asks, and the next Sunday I open my front door to Bevan and Rob, guitar in hand. Guitar-playing lawyers all know each other.

Soon the three of us are playing an eclectic mix of folk, country and rock music together every week. Rob and Bevan do the dishes after dinner, while I read to Jakob and tuck him into bed. Afterwards, we play and sing until late. Bevan sings melody, I sing harmony and they take turns to play Miss Martin, as we call my father's old Martin guitar, named for her curvaceous shape. It's the first time outside work that I have meaningful relationships with men that aren't romantic. It feels easy, relaxing and fun.

"What have you done to your foot?" Rob exclaims in alarm as I rise to make coffee one night.

Although it's summer, I wear black opaque tights under my cotton floral summer dress to hide my lumpy leg and big foot.

"Nothing. I was born that way," I say

And seeing I don't invite discussion, neither he nor Bevan ask again. It's the way I still handle every inquiry – the way my mother taught me. Over the years, my leg has maintained its shape, and while the severed nerves from the operations give me regular electric shocks and my foot still swells in summer and with overuse, it rarely gives me serious trouble. The scars finally healed, along with my fear of rejection. I have a lumpy leg and a big fat square foot, but I also have a son, a job, a flat (with a big fat mortgage) – and a life with words and music – just as I wished for when I was married to Danny and bought the little talisman of the medieval lute player.

Rik is moving to Traralgon, two hours' drive away, to be with his new girlfriend, an older woman with two teenagers. Jakob is five and at school. I worry about the long drive and how he'll fit into this new family, with this new mother, a stranger. Is she kind? Will she welcome my son? Rik had asked me the same questions when I'd blithely married on the rebound, a marriage that failed. I worry about the many changes in my son's young life and the damage that may have been done by us all.

It's a relief when, despite travelling between our two families, Jakob remains sunny, curious, and talkative and seems to enjoy being part of this new family in Traralgon. On Friday nights, when it's my weekend to have him, we continue our tradition of sitting up in bed watching musicals and eating lollies, and whenever I get free tickets to anything we go to shows.

"What are they doing?" he asks when we sit in the Princess Theatre one night watching Frank N Furter and Janet writhe under a blanket during *The Rocky Horror Show*.

"Playing!" I say, making a mental note to check the rating on any future shows.

He's spending that Easter with Rik in Traralgon. It's the first Easter I'll spend alone – no longer part of Danny's family, no longer part of Rik's and far away from Mum and Walter, who've moved to an old Victorian house in Maldon, two hours' drive away.

"Will you come and visit me?" she asked before the move. "Of course, I will," I said, and I did, bringing Jakob on the school holidays.

But the distance means most of our communication is limited to my weekly phone calls, where I report my son's progress and she dispenses encouragement: "You do so much for him!" she says.

I'm used to spending nights alone in our flat with my guitar while Jakob sleeps, but with everyone else doing family things, Good Friday to Easter Tuesday feels like a canyon of time to fill. Bevan is away. I wonder what Rob's doing. We get along well musically, but I don't know much about him personally. Will he think it weird if I invite him over for a jam without Bevan? What do I have to lose? Only a few lonely nights. I pick up the phone.

"Are you free for a jam?"

"Sure. Why don't you come over here?" he says.

He lives with a friend in Hawthorn. We play and sing for a while and then walk down Glenferrie Road to pick up a pizza. He's a country boy. Like me, he moved around a lot as a child, as his father was a stock and station agent, charged with reviving ailing offices before moving on to the next office in the next town. With his furrowed brow and slightly rotund figure, Rob seems kind and wise.

"How old are you?" I ask, as we sit at his kitchen table with pizza and wine.

"Twenty-six."

I nearly fall off my chair. It doesn't matter. We're just playing music together. The next week we meet again for dinner – and regularly after that, between jamming with Bevan.

Months later, worried that our late-night playing might offend my downstairs neighbour, I suggest we all go to Mum and Walter's in Maldon for a winter weekend of music. "Bring the guitar," has become her new mantra. I'm too shy to play for anyone, but I feel fortified by Bevan and Rob.

Rob blinks when Mum greets us at the door, heavily made up, her dyed black hair matching her black pants, a rope of red beads diving into the suntanned neckline of her white shirt.

"I know which one you like," she says, as Rob and Bevan go off to the spare bedroom to digest the extravagant meal she's provided. I don't comment. I know which one I like too. And why.

Between the Easter weekend and that weekend at Mum's, Rob came over for another jam. After a few songs, we abandoned our guitars and found ourselves sitting on the bed. I was nervous. I was 33 and had a child. My body was different now, and there was my leg. Rob's blue-grey eyes and his furrowed brow were unflinching as I explained my scars.

"I guess that means I'll have to love it even more," he said.

18

A month later, I hand Rob a hefty swag of paper. "I've photocopied a few of my stories for you," I say. In my history of serial marriage, my work was largely ignored by Danny and derided by Rik. I'm keen for Rob to meet the other me: the person I am at work. My friends smiled approvingly when he eruditely and succinctly talked about history and politics. I assume he will be interested in the type of politics I write about.

He doesn't read them. He pretends to, making a few stammering comments when I ask. But I can tell he hasn't really. I'm disappointed. I puzzle over it, but don't comment, not wanting to push him away.

Instead, I invite him to the next Accent lunch at the Southern Cross hotel, celebrating Accent's 25th birthday. The title of the lunch is *Great Expectations – Generations of Change*. The speakers include Dr Helen Randell, director of the Council for Adult Education, journalist and comedienne, Wendy Harmer, writer journalist Helen Garner and quirky artist Mirka Moira, who proves her point about not wearing a bra by lifting up her shirt to reveal all, which tickles Rob.

"It was like a feminist rally," he laughs later. I'm disappointed again. How can I be with someone who trivialises my work? I know that's not his intention. He just doesn't seem to get it.

He's not the only one. Every Wednesday morning, when Accent is published, ABC broadcaster Terry Lane confesses to getting "terribly upset". On air one morning, he suggests that to stop Accent spoiling his day with its outrageous generalisations about men, his wife should remove it from the paper and burn it. One particular story, about a fireman rescuing a toddler who got his head stuck between some railings in a shop incensed him. The female reporter wrote that men didn't generally appear to be as kind or empathetic as women, "but this didn't mean they weren't kind at all".

Terry takes it to mean they aren't kind at all and rages on air against these "preposterous and outrageous generalisations".

To set him straight, I offer a challenge. He can interview me on air, if I can interview him off air. The bravado I feel when I issue the challenge evaporates once I'm sitting beside him in the ABC studios in Melbourne. My mouth goes dry. I can hardly form my words. "Can I please have a drink of water?" I squeak, after I object to the generalisations he's made about feminists when he calls them "the boiler-suit brigade".

"Well, what should I call them?" he demands in exasperation.

The question perplexes and infuriates me. Don't women deserve the same attribution and respect as men?

"By their names," I say.

"That was fantastic," Rob says when we discuss it later. He was sitting in his car listening and whooped in delight when he heard it. His comment gives me confidence for my interview with Terry a few days later – and for our relationship in future.

But in the following weeks it's Rob, not me, who seems less sure about whether we should be together. He has to go to a legal conference in Adelaide. Can he make a decision when he returns? I'm anxious, but I understand. It's a big decision to be the partner of an older woman with a child. I wait for him at the airport on his return, scanning his face for clues. I've made a decision of my own. I want to be with him. Not because I'm afraid of being alone, but because he makes my life better. It feels like a decision based on something real, not imagined. I hope he feels the same way.

He does.

"You've got definition," he tells me, as he holds my hand later in my flat.

Definition? What does it mean? Perhaps I've passed some sort of test?

"It means … substance," he says.

Later, when I think about it, I realise it's probably the greatest compliment I've ever received from a man. The women I write about for Accent are women of substance; women like Dame Phyllis Frost, Senator Janine Haines, Victoria's first premier Joan Kirner, and US feminist authors Susan Faludi and Naomi Wolf. It means they are women who must be taken seriously, who can't be easily cast aside. In the years since Rik and I parted, despite my brief marital detour, I'd pulled myself together through work and the joys and demands of parenthood. I'd lost, but also gained. I was a woman of substance.

* * *

Two months later the flat across the hallway from me becomes available and Rob moves in.

"You're not my father," Jakob says the following Saturday, as he waits with Rob at the market while I rush off to buy meat, and he stands on Rob's toes to show him he means it. Rob doesn't try to be his father. Rik's already fulfilling that role. It's enough to let me be the mother. Rob and Jakob play board games together and become friends.

When the lease on his flat ends, we have to make a decision. Should we stop paying double rent and get a place together? Should we – dare I say it, get married? (Should I, dare I say it, *keep* getting married!) I am 35. Old. He's 28. Young. What if he wants children of his own? I worry my body will let me down, punishing me for all those babies I didn't want. We decide to have the honeymoon first in Tasmania. If that proves fruitful, we'll marry.

Months go by. No fruit.

"Let's test you first," the obstetrician says, when I explain my strange symptoms, which I fear are menopausal.

Rob is stunned and tearful when I tell him the good news. "We'd better get married then," he says quietly.

"We's a bit sick of weddings," Mum says in a small baby voice when I call her.

I am stung. Doesn't she realise this is the real thing?

PART THREE

Finding

19

Three years after Rob and I marry, my mother finds a new mantra. She's no longer alone with "nothing and no one". She's 67 and mortal. "Tis but 'a short dance across the stage'," she chants ominously.

The phrase is a reduction of the quote from Macbeth: *Life's but a walking shadow, a poor player that struts and frets his hour upon the stage, and then is heard no more.*

I assume it's these feelings of mortality that make her want to contact my sister again after a 21-year estrangement.

"She is my daughter," Mum says, dismissing my astonished look. "Do you think I should do it?"

"Maybe. You've got nothing to lose," I say, but I know she does. If Julie refuses, Mum will surely regard it as further proof that my sister "had chosen HIM", my father, opening old wounds. As a teenager, it never occurred to me that Mum would want to contact Julie again – she'd had nothing good to say about her. But now, as a mother myself, I understand that such bonds don't really break. They become wounds – and my mother is anxious to heal.

Despite her fear of rejection, she enlists my help. I ring Tess for Julie's address and Mum writes a cautious letter, inviting her to meet for lunch. I'm amazed when my sister agrees – and that the meeting is cordial. They agree to keep in touch.

"It would be nice if you could write her a letter to tell her you were happy about it," Mum says. "I always hoped you could be friends one day."

Really? Am I happy about it? I'm not sure. I haven't seen Julie for 16 years – not since my brief visit to hospital after the birth of her daughter. It's been 21 years since we had any meaningful contact. Over the years I've made sisters of all my female friends. Did I need the sister who was always a disrupter to come back into my life?

"You're very different. She's very hard," Mum reminds me, as if her relationship with my sister can only be understood in relation to me.

I have new family now: Rob, our two-year old daughter Greta and Jakob, who is now 10. Rob's parents are devoted Nana and Pa, and Mum and Walter are Grandma and Grandpa – distant emotionally as well as geographically.

"It was surprisingly easy to write," I confide to Tess when I mention the letter I finally write to my sister. "But it was bloody hard to post. It's still in my bag."

A few weeks later, on a cool Saturday morning in autumn, I sit in the quiet and pretty tearooms at Tecoma, near our home in Upwey in the Dandenong Ranges, looking through the white lattice window for the stranger that's my sister, wondering what we'll have in common after all these years. I know from Mum that she is divorced, and has reverted to her maiden name, which to me feels like a feminist act. She's also reclaimed her full name – Juliana. I'm glad. I've always admired that beautiful name, although I find it hard to think of her as anyone other than Julie, the sister of my childhood. She's left the chemist shop and trained as a counsellor, which impresses me. Beyond that I know little about her.

I have no doubt she knows about me – if she reads *The Age*. Not only do I have the perfect family, I'm famous for it. I was eight months pregnant when, in a bid to increase female readership, Alan Kohler *The Age* editor asked me to write a column called *A New Life Journal*, about my baby's first year. I planned to change our names, but just as it felt inauthentic to change the names in the too-truthful play I wrote as a teenager, I used our real names in the column, pouring out our family's trials and tribulations each week, accompanied by not-too-flattering cartoons of us all.

Rob doesn't mind. He rarely reads the column and only objects to his image when a colleague sticks a clipping on his office door. His lack of interest irks me, but I've long come to realise Rob doesn't read anything much, apart from what's required for work. He's an audio guy. Radio is his main source of information. It doesn't matter. I have plenty of other readers, mostly new mothers like me.

"Your life so often mirrors my own," they write. By the end of the first year, I receive so many letters that when a woman stops us in the street one day, Jakob waves goodbye with the words, "Bye, fan!"

That's it. I end the column and close the door on our family life – reluctantly reclaiming it a year later after *The Age* appoints me Family and Society Reporter. Few "family stories" ever make it past the back pages and I feel typecast. Juggling work and child care from our home in Upwey proves impossible. It's easier to work from home, writing about my own family again in a new column called Family Postcard.

I wonder if my sister reads it. I hope not.

* * *

The shop doorbell tinkles. I look up. She's smaller than I remember, with fair skin like Mum, blonde hair layered and teased, wearing huge rose-gold narrow hoop earrings, jeans and a black slim-line short jacket. On her wrist, which is daintier than mine, she wears a heavy rose-gold chain bracelet. Her wide-spaced amber-green eyes are separated by something I don't recognise – a pert turned-up nose – and her teeth are white and even.

"I nearly didn't come," she confesses as she sits down. I chatter nervously about being nervous too.

"You sound so posh," she says, making me self-conscious. My accent is far from the standard that Mum once set for us, yet here's another thing that sets us apart.

She confesses she had a nose job and her teeth fixed as soon as she could afford it. My nose is the least of my worries. I don't tell her about my leg job. I rarely speak about it with anyone, least of all a sister I barely know.

Curiosity makes us both charming and forgiving, as between tea and scones we begin to pass each other pieces of the missing puzzle that we've both kept over the years. She has a new partner, Macca, a builder, and she works in the payroll department at a funeral home and as a part-time bereavement counsellor and plans to study Social Work.

After she tells me about her life, I tell her about mine, including all the bad bits. I'm not looking for pity. It's a form of protection against the "good girl" image Mum always held up to my sister. That was then. I want Julie to see me as I am now, so I tell her about the rocky road that led me to this Nirvana – the marriages, the abortions and the pain. I don't mention work, except in a jokey way, telling how when Rob lost his job due to Government budget cuts after Greta was born, Mum told me to stop being angry and use my intelligence, and I took her advice and used my influence with Attorney General Jan Wade to help Rob get a new job. I know I'm boasting, contradicting my efforts to appear unworthy of envy, but I can't help wanting my sister to admire me a little.

Juliana stares at me, her big eyes even bigger. And then she tells me about her pain. How her diabetes medication interfered with her birth control and she found herself pregnant. Dad and her husband Peter, suddenly pious, invoked their Catholic upbringing and persuaded her to keep the baby. Juggling work and motherhood was a challenge. Eventually the marriage failed and she left.

"I'm not like Dad. I'm good with money. I always make sure I have 'piss-off money'," she says.

It's my turn to stare. I'm not good with money. I'm more inclined to use it to escape into marriage. I find myself admiring her foresight and resilience. I didn't want a baby at the age of 23 either. I wonder how I would have coped if I hadn't had a choice.

I show her photos of my son and daughter and she laughs when I tell her Jakob was best man at my wedding to Rob and my friend Carolyn had to keep altering the dress as I was pregnant with Greta, and had ballooned out to size 20 by the time we married in a small Italian restaurant in North Fitzroy. Five months later, Greta was born – on Jakob's birthday.

"How'd you manage that?"

"She had to be induced two weeks early as my leg was affected. He asked if it could be on his birthday. The gift that keeps on giving."

We laugh together, like two close girlfriends meeting for lunch – or two sisters.

"Do you see Mum and Walter much?" she finally asks. In the hour we've been talking, I haven't mentioned Mum and she hasn't mentioned Dad.

"They come twice a year on the train, on cheap Tuesdays, which means the kids have to have a day off school. It's like a Royal Visit," I say. "Do you see much of Dad?"

She nods. He's a devoted "Pa" to her daughter, now 16. She shows me a photo of a striking girl with fair skin, dark hair and Dad's bright blue eyes. After 10 years of marriage, Doris and Dad had separated and he was building himself a new house in Geelong, she says.

I'm not surprised they've separated. Dad was never easy to live with.

"He was jealous of Pam and Pip," Juliana says "Dad didn't like them being there."

Pam and Pip, Doris's youngest children, were close to Doris before she and Dad married. I could imagine how such jealousy must have rankled.

"Dottie was good for Dad. She supported him to do the things he wanted to do," Juliana says. I hope she didn't tell Mum this, which feels like another betrayal.

"He's writing you a letter," she says.

A letter? I'm not sure I want a letter. Our previous two reunions were disappointing. I smile and nod, not wanting to appear discouraging.

Without comment, she takes out a small black zip-up purse and removes a tiny tube with a pin on the end. Expertly, she pricks her finger, testing the small drop of blood that appears, writes down a number and, gathering a pinch of flesh between her thumb and forefinger from under her shirt, injects herself. I've never seen a diabetic injecting themselves before.

"Macca and I are getting married on the Isle of Mann in Scotland, where his family originally came from," she says as she returns the needle to the purse. "I haven't found a dress yet."

I grin. "You can have mine. Come to the house now and have a look." It seems like the perfect solution. After all, I have a few to choose from.

***

It has to be cut down to fit, but she takes the cream lace Mariana Hardwick three-quarter length lace dress with a sweetheart neckline that I wore for my second failed marriage in San Francisco. We have the same taste in dresses, if not husbands.

"I've got Dad's old guitar," I say. She looks surprised, and I wonder why Dad didn't offer it to her. I show her how it's been fixed and we sing a couple of the old songs our parents sang, marvelling at how we remember the words. As we make plans to meet again, it occurs to me that my readers, who are my surrogate family, should meet my long-lost sister.

"How would you like to write a column about our reunion with me?" I ask.

20

We meet at my place in Upwey a month later so I can tape the interview. She brings a bottle of brandy and a bottle of diet Coke. I buy a cask of white wine. Conscious that she's entering my world, I let her start.

"Ready?"

She nods and I press play.

"This is a real Family Postcard," she says. "This is Jane's real family, not her extended family. This is Jane's root family."

She leans into the microphone. "Juliana Cafarella here in her own right. I am not an extension of Jane. I am an individual."

"She looks suspicious," I say into the microphone.

"She feels suspicious," she says, eyeing me. "You can't trust these journalists, even if they are family."

So why are you doing this?

"Because Jane's written so much other crap about her family she may as well put a bit of truth in it," she says. "Meet the rest of Jane's family."

So, she has read the columns. I am almost too truthful about my family life with Rob, but the 600 weekly words are in their own way a construct. Has she seen through this? Apparently.

"I feel sorry for your family. You ridicule them a lot in the paper," she says. "I looked at it and thought poor Rob. She's exploiting her family."

"You're next," I quip.

"See! I made one simple statement. You can twist it with two words and now it's got a different connotation to it," she says accusingly.

She pours another brandy. I pour another wine.

In all these years we'd been separated did she ever think of me?

"No," she says. "It was just me and Dad. It was easier that way."

I nod. I hadn't thought of her either. So what made her agree to meet?

"Maturity," she says.

Macca was close to his family, which made her wonder about hers. "And because I'd met Mum." She pauses, looking at me. "If you shut the book before the end, you only have half the story."

Meeting me has been a breeze compared to meeting Mum, she says, sipping her brandy. She worried about what to wear, how to speak, what she'd look like.

"It was just horrible. I took brandy with me. When I saw her walking up the street all that went (the feelings of insecurity, not the brandy!)." What were you expecting?

"A nice old lady. A grandma type. A nice, nurturing gentle mother."

(What planet was she on?)

What did you see?

"Somebody like they were in drag. I thought, ooh I've got nothing to worry about."

I feel a pang. My sister sees a drag queen. I see a woman desperately trying to hide her age and herself behind a mask.

But did you remember her as a nice old lady?

"I remembered her as a bitch," she says.

I startle. Mum was difficult, but a bitch?

"She sent me a pressure cooker for a wedding present," she says. "I didn't even open it, I thought she's trying to kill me."

Really? I think of all the nights when we were kids, when Mum came home from work and wearily threw a cheap cut of meat and some tomatoes and onions into the pressure cooker for a quick meal. To me, the gift of a pressure cooker showed she understood the sort of pressure her daughter was under as a working woman. But to have a future together, my sister and I have to agree on a version of the past.

"I really believed she contacted me because she was dying," Juliana says. "… this was part of her guilt trip, so she could die in peace."

Of course, our mother isn't dying – despite her many illnesses. But my estranged sister couldn't imagine any other reason for Mum wanting to contact her again. Even then, she hesitated.

A visit to Nana Cafarella's grave changed her mind. "There was this spirit, saying 'You have to make the family complete. Unless you put the pieces together, it's not going to work.'"

"How did you feel when you met me?" I ask, confident that I'll fare better than Mum, The Drag Queen.

"I hated you when we were kids," Juliana said. "Mum and Dad made us compete. You were brainier, you were gentler, you fitted into the clone and I didn't."

I nod, ignoring the sting of the word "hate" while marvelling at her fearlessness. I'm wary of offending her, but she doesn't seem worried about offending me,

"I was shocked when I met you," she says. "You were more woggy-looking than I thought. You're a lot like Dad."

Like Dad? Not only was I like Dad, she was like Mum, she says.

"They got the wrong ones," she says, and her wide-spaced amber-green eyes stare at me in exactly the same way as Mum's.

"I think I'm more like Mum because I didn't like being a mother," she says. "I think Mum understood but would never say."

This feels true. Mum will never admit this to Juliana because they aren't close, but she's always had plenty to say about it to me: "There I was stuck in a bad marriage with ill-health and two sick children."

My sister, who feels both strange and familiar, pours another brandy and Coke and looks at me shrewdly. "I think you're two people. You're the journalist, and you're the mother, and confused about which you want to be.

"You're good at twisting things around, like Dad," she says, analysing me. "You're good with words. You make things sound justifiable, realistic, and it sounds like the truth coming out of his mouth. But you have to practise what you preach. I think you and Dad will get along very well because you'll have some bitey things to get in depth about, whereas Dad and I fight."

Her words feel both true and mean. Over the years, I've also observed that, like Dad, I'm good with words. I also enjoy drawing and playing guitar. If I'm a manipulator, why did she agree to this interview?

She shrugs. "I said to Macca, 'I liked her'. And that surprised me, because as a kid I felt I had to compete with her. Now the choice is mine."

She looks up, studying me further.

"I was surprised at how honest you were. I thought you'd be more guarded and tentative about the conversation."

Why is she agreeing to such honesty being in print?

"Because it's part of Jane's postcard from nowhere."

So, you don't mind?

"If you don't twist it, I won't mind."

***

I twist it. I have to. I cut all the stuff about Mum, which I know will blow up the new bridge we've had all tentatively crossed. My sister's comments are both insulting and perceptive.

She took control and I let her, too curious and too afraid to frighten her away.

A few months later I receive my father's letter. The tone is cordial, polite, cautious and benign. He's happy Juliana and I have met. Perhaps we can meet, too?

It's been nine years since our previous failed meeting. I planned to be furious at this request for another meeting. And I am: furious that I'm strangely touched that the man who always fled is prepared to stay and try again. We haven't always been enemies. For a brief period, in the years we'd lived at Heslop Street, Parkdale, he'd claimed me as his work mate and fellow dreamer. Perhaps, after all these years, we can claim each other?

"I'm supposed to be angry with you, you bastard," I reply.

I warn him – I have questions. My reunion with Juliana has been confronting. The journalist in me has begun to question my mother's version of the family story. What's my father's version? How and why did my parents really get together? Who is the mysterious Perry who lured him into the milk bar business, and did he really go to jail? What role did the bankruptcy play in the failure of their marriage and how does anyone go bankrupt twice? And, above all, how did my father end up with Doris? Were they having an affair all along, as my mother had come to suspect?

I don't elaborate in the letter. I will save that for our meeting. I hope he'll recognise me.

"Perhaps we can compare our aching backs as well as our aching hearts?" I write, signing it: "Your daughter, Jane."

A week later, he replies: "Thanks for the title (BASTARD). It broke me up and can I say, WELL SAID."

He promises to answer my questions truthfully. He has nothing to hide.

"Failings I have many, but NOBODY'S PERFECT, and I am NOBODY," he writes, which feels both clever and sad. Juliana is right. He's good at twisting words. Like me. His purpose isn't to "turn the tide" about my side of the story but to "stem the flow" and get some interaction with me, he says.

"I've never been scared of meeting you. TERRIFIED is a better word. Wear a white carnation in case we may walk past each other."

Terrified? Of me? It suggests remorse, and that he's changed since our last meeting when he didn't recognise me or bother to ask about my son.

Meeting Juliana makes me wonder if we are all that different after all. Amongst the joy of discovering each other, we discover a mutual love of musicals. As a celebration gift, she buys us tickets to *Beauty and the Beast* and *The Hunchback of Notre Dame* – both musicals about outcasts reclaimed, although neither of us realises it then. Perhaps we are all outcasts? Her words from our interview feel true: "If you shut the book before the end, you only have half the story."

21

He doesn't look terrified. He's already seated in front of a cup of coffee, smoking and flicking through a magazine when I arrive at the Old Paper Shop Deli in South Melbourne.

"You look older. You've put on a bit of weight," he says, eyeing me, as I sit opposite.

He's put on weight too. He's 62, shorter and heavier set than I remember. His hair has receded and is thin and grey. He looks like the man he most hates in the world: his father. But I know better than to tell him that.

"What have you been doing all these years?" I say, as an icebreaker for my real questions.

"Working three days a week, driving cabs," he says, blowing a ring of smoke towards me. "But I never paid any tax. I drove under the boss's name."

He's always worked in multiple jobs under false names to avoid paying tax, but it seems strange to remind me of it now.

Driving cabs is easier than running the newsagency he and Doris once owned near Geelong, he says.

"All the kids used to come in and read the porn. I was always chasing them out."

After that he had a hardware business. Between driving taxis, he's building himself a new house in Conneware, also near Geelong.

As he picks up his coffee with his right hand, my eyes linger on the left. The flap crafted from the skin from his left thigh has browned with age, and is folded clumsily over his fingerless fist like a piece of over-cooked leftover pastry.

"You're finding that hard to look at," he says.

"No," I say lowering my eyes. Why do I stare? I hate it when people stare at my foot.

"It's fucking ugly," he says, as if answering my question.

"Juliana said you and Doris had split up," I say, planning to lead into the question of how they got together in the first place.

He nods. "I got sick of it being all about her family. I thought what about my family." (Indeed.)

The closeness between Doris and Pip especially bothered him. "They'd be sitting up in bed together talking. They even did a chocolate-making course together. It was unnatural."

Unnatural? I think of the many times I've sat up in bed talking with my own children – something I've never done with him or Mum. It seems natural that as a young widow, Doris gathered her children around her, and that this carried over into their adult lives. I wonder whether this reunion, like all the others, is a mistake.

It isn't just my cousins who came between him and Doris, he says

"There's God, the Pope and then Doris."

She was a pillar of the local Anglican Church, which gave him "the shits".

"I spent 20 years with one sister and 10 years with the other," he says, as if he's talking about prison sentences, not marriages. I imagine my cousins Pam and Pip are relieved the marriage is over. I wish we could compare notes.

He's changed his name back to Cafarella to mark the occasion. Caff was too confusing and didn't change his luck. "Everyone thought it was Cap or Cat."

He doesn't ask why I never changed my name. If he did, I'd tell him it's a feminist act, not paternal pride. He doesn't ask why I sign my cartoons CAF either. He probably doesn't know about them.

We pick up our coffee cups and put them down. The waiter begins putting chairs on tables. Closing time. This isn't the conversation I imagined. He said he'd answer my questions, yet he offers no invitation to ask them. The journalist in me doesn't need an invitation, but the anxious daughter does.

Finally, he offers a question of his own.

"I hear Rob's a lawyer?"

I sigh. I know what's coming: the question everyone with a lawyer in the family is always asked.

"I've got a legal problem he might be able to help me with."

"He's not in private practice," I say, wondering if this is the real reason he's agreed to meet.

He explains the problem anyway; some dodgy deal he's involved with. I explain again why Rob can't help.

Silence.

"I've heard your son is very musically talented?"

"Yes," I say, grateful for a new topic, and I tell him how Tess had shown Jakob some simple tunes on her new baby grand piano when he was nine, and how on the way home he had said, "I have to learn piano", as if it was a need not a whim.

"Tess is the only piano teacher I know who never plays the piano," Dad says, diverting the conversation from praise of a grandson to criticism of a sister.

The questions that hang heavy in my mind float lightly away as we pay and head out.

"Did you drive or come by train?" I ask.

"Drove," he said. "I'm doing up an old Citroen."

Unlike other cars, the Citroen is suspended on bags of oil, he says. That's what makes it such a smooth ride.

"I can never work out what colour it is," he says, pointing proudly to what looks like a low-slung small spaceship parked nearby.

I look. "Mushroom."

"That's exactly right," he says, and for the first time he looks impressed.

"How do you manage driving, with your hand?"

"I've made a little wooden knob on the left side of the steering wheel to help me steer," he says, and I have a sudden memory of watching him steer with his knees while rolling a cigarette when I am a child.

"You'll have to come to Upwey to meet the family," I say, as the afternoon sun sinks and we part. I'm glad when he agrees. The truth isn't lost, merely postponed.

"Grandpa Frank is coming," I tell Greta, a month later. She's excited – until she sees his hand and runs off screaming. She's used to my "rukky reg", as she calls my leg, but this is too much, despite the Barbie doll he brings her.

Jakob is less disturbed. He plays piano for him. I show him his old guitar, and tell him how it brought Rob and I together, and Rob plays it for him. I'm still too shy. I make lunch. It's show and tell, but not in the way I'd imagined.

"You'll have to come to Conneware," he says, as he leaves. "But the house isn't finished."

* * *

It takes me three hours to drive from Boronia to my father's house in Conneware a month later to get the answers to the questions that aren't finished either. The real question I am asking myself is deeper: is my father really the "Gigolo" and the villain my mother always made out?

I leave three hours later, without challenging him. The house he's building is a replica of all the houses I've grown up in – a mess of tools, paint tins, splattered drop sheets, car parts, dirty clothes, festering food, boxes and junk.

"I cleaned up for you," he jokes, as he leads me to the kitchen. As soon as he's finished, it will be featured in "worser homes and gardens" he says, referring to the popular magazine *Better Homes and Gardens*, and he tells me about the special stove he'll (never) put in the kitchen and the cupboards he'll (never) build.

"Sorry about the heating," he says pointing to a large industrial gas bottle with a roaring blue flame near an old reclining chair, and I marvel that he hasn't blown himself up, as I recall how he always fell asleep with a half-smoked cigarette burning in a nearby ashtray when I was a child.

He has to get the house to lock-up stage before he can get council approval to sell it and use the money to retire. But he's having trouble with his hips. "What used to take me six weeks now takes six months."

Juliana warned me he lived in a mess – and rarely let anybody in the house to see it. He's clearly embarrassed by it and I'm embarrassed for him.

"Thanks for lunch, Dad," I say, as I leave. My mother was wrong: he wasn't a villain after all. She was also right: he was a fool.

Our relationship reverts to occasional phone calls. He calls, usually at dinner time, asking about the family and cuts me off as I answer, before vomiting up his day on me. Until one day in exasperation, I cut him off with a question of my own.

"What prompted you to finally separate from Mum?" I ask, hoping to lead to the question of what had prompted him to hook up with Doris.

"Well, that was your fault," he says.

I gasp. "My fault?"

"You were the messenger," he says. "I would never have left your mother. I was too much of a traditional Italian. She wanted a trial separation and I agreed. Then she sent you around asking about a solicitor."

I was indeed the unwitting messenger, standing on the veranda at Wavertree in Heslop Street at the age of 17 with a yellow envelope and my mother's instruction: "Tell your father I want a divorce." But hardly at fault.

"I was a child being manipulated," I stammer.

"I'm not blaming you, but you were the messenger," he repeats. "You were always on your mother's side," he says, explaining why he never contacted me afterwards.

I find an excuse to hang up so I can absorb this accusation. It's true. As a child, I was on my mother's side. But I wasn't responsible for the unhappiness that made her want to leave.

I don't hear from my father again, nor do I contact him. More than ever, I am on my mother's side. Since she reconnected with my sister, we have all embraced the normality we missed out on for all those years. Christmases and Easters are spent together at Maldon. A splendid cook and hostess, she is as perfectly presented as the dishes she serves.

"Come for a walk with us," I say, once. She shakes her head. "I have to wash the lettuce."

Between charming and cooking for their many friends, she travels to Europe with Walter several times, and takes up oil painting – still life with fruit, copies of famous paintings, and her favourite – a portrait of Walter, looking unusually relaxed and happy, painted from a photo snapped with friends.

But gradually, the effort of maintaining the house with its wood-fired heaters and large garden becomes too much for Walter and they move to Castlemaine 30 minutes from Maldon, to be "closer to the hospital".

Juliana and Macca move too, to nearby Newbridge to realise their dream of a hobby farm, and Rob and I move to Boronia, closer to high school for Jakob. We want Mum and Walter to consider moving to Boronia to be closer to us in future, so we can care for them as they age. I've finally paid off my debt to Walter, but not my debt of gratitude.

"We're not ready for the nursing home yet," Mum says, adding, "Nobody cares about you in the suburbs."

"We do," I say which only upsets her further.

Her comment feels like a repeat of the "nothing and no one" comments of my adolescence – a refusal to acknowledge my presence and my love.

"Children leave," she warns, when I press her, citing examples of friends who've moved near their children, only to have them pack up and move to another state or even another country.

It's not her rejection of my invitation to be closer that hurts and puzzles me; it's her fury, especially when she cancels our impending visit.

"Why couldn't she just say, 'Thank you, but we're not ready yet'?" I ask Rob.

"They don't understand you're being generous," he says.

They don't seem to understand why we want to visit them in their new home either.

"It's too far", "You're too busy" or "Walter's got a doctor's appointment on Monday", Mum says. Whenever I call, she is just coming in or going out.

"It's chaos here. We're frantic. One day when you're retired, you'll understand how busy it is," she says.

In a fury of my own I call her and tell her I'm sick of feeling like an imposition, citing everything from her refusal to see us, to her constant references to being stuck in a bad marriage with sick children when I was a child. Throughout my childhood and adolescence, the world was presented to me through her eyes. Now I was looking through my own. All I want is what other people have: a parent who welcomes them.

The next day, I write her a regretful but frank letter, explaining that "one day your small dance across the stage will be over and it will be too late".

More fury. "I very quickly moved from 'Mother Extraordinaire' to 'Bottom of the RUBBISH TIP!'" she writes in reply. "Goodbye. I will not sign Mum, as in your eyes I have never been one."

A letter from Walter follows: "Your mother was devastated by your letter." They've spent a lot of money and time establishing their new life in Castlemaine and want to enjoy it while they are able, he explains.

It's useless to try to explain that our suggestion is a gesture of goodwill, not an attack, so I apologise – with flowers and a note – saying I look forward to visiting them in their new home.

"Where will you stay?" Mum asks, when I ring to fix a date. They've turned the second bedroom into a grand dining room. We stay at Celestine House, in nearby Guildford, and visit them for lunch.

"How come we can't sit at that table?" Jakob asks, pointing to the elegantly set dining table in the elegant dining room as he perches on a stool next to me and Rob at the kitchen table, while Greta balances on a cane chair beside him, boosted by cushions.

"That's for visitors tomorrow," Mum says.

The new smaller garden in Castlemaine includes a small statue of an angel – Possum's grave. Shortly before they moved, Mum found her rigid under a chair in the lounge room at Maldon, dead from a heart attack. Mum was heartbroken. They bought another dog – a small black and white Papillion with big fluffy ears, whom Mum named Lulu – my childhood nickname, from my middle name Louise. But they weren't used to the mess and disruption of a puppy and before any real attachment could form, they gave it away.

That year I'm turning 40. "You know the rule. We don't give presents on your birthday and all. Does that still stand?" Mum says when I ring her and mention the small celebration we are having.

"Of course."

The no-present policy is both a relief and a disappointment, as she always complains about the effort of choosing it and posting it. But lately, I've begun to resent it, not because I want presents but because it feels like another symptom of her reluctance to engage.

My sister ignores the no-present policy, arriving with food, drink, flowers – never empty-handed – embarrassing Mum into giving us all $20 for "a bottle of vino", for birthdays thereafter.

"Why did she bring all this stuff? I told her not to," Mum complains to me after Juliana leaves each family gathering. I'm the only one who witnesses Mum's true feelings, which I never challenge, leaving me feeling guilty and remorseful but unable to break this triangle. Once when Juliana has surgery on her finger – a complication of diabetes – she drops by Castlemaine on the way home, just as I'm visiting Mum.

"You look nice," Mum says, greeting her with a kiss.

As we say goodbye and the door closes, she says, "Didn't she look terrible? It's all that drinking."

Juliana carries a bottle of brandy and diet coke wherever she goes. Mum carries a glass of "vino", but she is genteel enough to wait till 5pm, the traditional cocktail hour. Alcohol makes my face red, so I can control my drinking. I'm a food-aholic, still following the spoon, which makes Mum's constant push for me to have second helpings feel like a goading comment on my weight.

"Have some more," she insists. "If you don't, I'll have to throw it all out."

I'm irritated but I can't help myself. I keep coming back for the food and the game we are all playing. So does Juliana. We both want something Mum can't or won't give – approval – although neither of us admit it to the other.

Above all, Juliana wants approval for the thing that's the most important to her – her work. The first time I visited her house I was struck by the dozens of small, framed certificates above her desk for all the short courses she'd done. After finishing her counselling course, she enrolled in university to study Social Work – although she called it "school", which felt like a diminishment, but perhaps it removed the fear.

"Why does she want to mix with THOSE people," Mum says when we're alone. "Those people" are the poor and disadvantaged, which to Mum means "no hopers".

"She was always attracted to the wrong kind."

"It's because they're the only people Juliana feels better than," my Aunt Tina observes, when, shocked at the cruelty of Mum's words, I repeat them to her. I know it's because Juliana identifies with "those people" – the people who can't do anything right.

University is a struggle. She left school at 15 and, apart from the many certificate courses, she had no formal education.

"Because you can write, I can't, because Mum always compared us and made us compete," she tells me, and as further proof, she adds indignantly: "Mum told me to ask you for help. She said you're writing a book."

I'm not. Not unless she means the book I edited for the Nursing Mother's Association of Australia, compiled from 30 years of information booklets, and which became a "breast seller".

"I thought you might write something someday," Mum tells me often, meaning The Great Australian Novel, not the Great Australian Boob Book. I don't have time. Between working, I'm too busy encouraging my own children's talents – piano for my son and singing for daughter – talents that Mum can understand.

When Juliana graduates with a Bachelor of Social Work, she's permitted to invite two guests to the ceremony. She chooses her husband Macca – and Dad.

"Why did she ask HIM? I was the ENCOURAGER," Mum says.

Walter echoes her outrage. "Your mother's very upset. She was the ENCOURAGER."

To Mum, it's further evidence of my sister's pathological disloyalty and perversity, exacerbated by the incident of the dog.

It's a cold Sunday afternoon. I'm sitting in my home office in Boronia, catching up on some work, when the phone rings.

"She came here with a dog," Mum says, her voice high with anxiety.

Like Mum, Juliana loves animals. Her new hobby farm in Newbridge is home to a menagerie of stray animals that would otherwise have been sausages or glue. But her key relationship is always with her dog. A dog doesn't just make a house a home; it makes life bearable. I know how she feels. When we move to Boronia, we acquire two dogs of our own – longhaired Chihuahuas called Bambi and Pepe – just like Possum – and a rabbit and a guinea pig and chooks. The whole suburban dream.

"You cannot impose a responsibility on someone, even if it's meant as a gift," Mum says, and she tells me she sent Juliana and the dog away.

My heart sinks. The incident of the dog has given my mother a new knife with which to stab an old wound.

"I can't do anything right," Juliana tells me later. She doesn't understand that two people in their 70s may not want the responsibility of a dog. For her, it represents all the rejection of her life.

True to her Cancer star sign, the crab, she retreats into her shell – remaining out of contact for weeks, and then gradually redefining the relationship on her terms. If she visits, it's briefly, on the way home from work, subtly provoking Mum by coming unannounced to the back door, to catch her off guard. She brings food to family events, even when she's asked not to, chatting charmingly to everyone except Mum. Her behaviour reminds me of when we were children and she scraped the new round-toed school shoes on the gravel to deliberately ruin them after Mum had refused to buy the more fashionable pointy-toed shoes.

And I'm in the middle. "Why is she like this?" Mum says, when we're alone, echoing her lament from my sister's adolescence

"She's a bitch," Juliana tells me whenever we meet for lunch, and the subject of Mum inevitably comes up.

Once or twice, I remind her of the books Mum bought us as children, the Pebbles dolls she saved up for at Christmas (modelled on the baby in the *Flintstones* cartoons), the birthday parties she organised with the many different flavours of Tarax bottles with their bobbing paper straws; the pavlovas and tea cakes she made, and the crummy jobs she worked so she could be there for us when we came home from school.

"I don't remember that," Juliana says.

It's no surprise that Juliana and Mum never got along, her husband Macca tells me. "She was raised by Frank."

"No, she wasn't," I say. "She lived with us until Mum and I left."

I don't count the year my sister spent in the convent.

"She told me that your Mum raised you and Frank raised her," Macca said, astounded. Emotionally yes, but we all lived together until they separated.

Soon after her 70th birthday, Mum is diagnosed with breast cancer and has a mastectomy. Armed with poetry books, flowers and cake, I visit her in Castlemaine Hospital, only to find her circled by friends, her chin trembling with pain as she charms and entertains them.

"Do you want me to send them away?" I whisper.

"I can't do that," she says, frowning at such an ungracious suggestion. The show must go on. She recovers but develops the habit of plucking the shirt from her chest, where it touches the raw scar, and every year she buys a daffodil broach from the Cancer Council to remind herself she survived.

Her brush with death fails to kill off her animosity towards my sister and the endless question of "Why is she like this?"

I want to scream: "She's like this, because you're like this, because you cast her in this role, just as you cast me in mine." But telling the truth will set me free in a way I can't handle. Hadn't my mother told me she could wipe me, just as she'd wiped my sister and Doris when I dared suggest I might visit my father after his fingers were severed all those years ago?

Mum has suffered yet another health blow with cancer, which may reoccur at any moment. There's no point in arguing. It's my job to understand. Except when I can't help myself.

"Have you heard from Juliana?" Mum asks when I call her a few weeks later at Easter.

"We've been emailing a bit," I say cautiously.

"She came here with all this wine and chocolate," Mum says in astonishment. "I told her we don't eat it anymore. I LOATHE it," she says, the word "loathe" landing like a wad of puke.

I'd heard the other side of this story. Rather than say thank you, Walter told Juliana they only drank Chardonnay, not Moselle, and as he was a Type 2 diabetic (although he never took any medication for it) he didn't eat chocolate, and that Mum preferred toffees. To ensure she didn't make the same mistake, he wrote down their preferred brands of wines and sweets.

"I was really angry, but I didn't show it," Juliana tells me later over lunch. "I got back in the car and said to Macca, I can't do anything right."

I'm angry too. I'm sick of these calls that demonise my sister. My mother has always cast us as opposites but our reunion has illuminated uncanny similarities. Apart from a mutual love of musicals, we discover that in the 21 years of our separation we've both bought paintings by the same artist, who turns out to be a friend of Doris's, we both have the same placemats and we both eat our favourite foods with a teaspoon to make them last longer – and we're both fed up with our mother.

"It's a pity you didn't see if for what it was," I tell Mum tersely.

There's a pause.

"What do you mean?" she asks.

"She hasn't spoken to you for a while, then she comes around bearing gifts. It's an olive branch."

"Well, she should know that we can't eat chocolate at our age," she says, and she repeats the incident of the dog.

I should have known. The only use my mother has for an olive branch is to hit my sister over the head with it.

"She didn't speak to us for months. What did she expect? Why is she like this? She always gets it wrong."

I'm getting it wrong too.

"I saw the milk bar story," Mum says, as a postscript, referring to a full-page story I've written for *The Age* about the failing milk bar industry. I'm pleased. Walter sometimes cuts out my stories, but Mum seldom comments.

"The whole of Castlemaine saw it," she says. "That's as far as you're allowed to go. You're not to write anything about me."

What? I wrote that our family once owned milk bars and that I worked in two as a teenager, but the story wasn't about Mum. How dare she invoke the ban she imposed when I wrote *The Triangle* play at the age of 17.

"It wasn't about you," I say. "It was about me and my memories. I'm entitled to write my own story."

And, emboldened by my sister's example, I hang up.

22

Bangkok, 2004

Khun Pakdee leans into the microphone, slipping easily from Thai to English, as he tells the audience at the Sukhothai Hotel what they've come to hear: the newly formed Metropolitan Opera of Bangkok is the first fully Thai opera company in the country.

The audience of diplomats, politicians and a princess or two, applauds and looks approvingly at the group of 20 or so singers, dressed in costume for a performance of excerpts from the Carl Maria Von Webber opera Der Freischutz – with Greta, aged 12 smiling in the front row. Fully Thai. With her olive skin and long straight dark hair parted in the centre, who knows that she's an imposter?

Just as Mum predicted that "children leave", six months earlier we had left Melbourne for Bangkok, where Rob had a new executive job – far away from our festering family relationships.

I am 48 – a year older than Mum was when she and Dad separated – and not counting my brief marital detour in San Francisco more than 15 years earlier, the furthest I've been is to the letter box and back to collect my freelance cheques. My son is at university in Perth, studying jazz composition and pursuing his own dreams. It's time for adventure – and to continue my dream to make my daughter a star, just as Momma Rose made her daughter Louise a star in one of my favourite musicals, Gypsy.

As soon as she could talk, Greta sang – in the pusher, in the car and the supermarket.

"Can you make her stop?" Jakob asked when he was a self-conscious teenager and she was still singing at the checkout one day. I didn't want her to stop. Heads were turning in the same way they turned when Mum sang. I was secretly thrilled by her confidence and her voice, which was rich and mature for her age. Jakob always drove his own talent, aided by his piano teacher, who recommended both the piano we bought and the high school he attended. But I drove hers. The day he left to go to Perth for uni, she threw herself on the lounge room floor in Boronia and wailed, "I want my brother!" To fill the void, I devoted myself to finding teachers and performance opportunities. Rob's long work hours, and the fact that I worked in my own freelance business from home threw us together in Melbourne in much the same way Mum and I were thrown together through illness and circumstance when I was a child, and casting myself as the ENCOURAGER, I drove her to rehearsals and lessons, until she became a star in a little constellation of her own, performing in amateur musicals and concerts.

I am determined to repeat her success in Bangkok – and so is she.

"I miss my friends. I miss Bambi and Pepe (our dogs) and singing," she sobs when we first arrive and find ourselves sitting together playing gin rummy with one-baht pieces in our new home in Samakee Place in the province of Nonthaburi, 30 kilometres from central Bangkok, as we wait for our shipment of furniture and personal belongings to arrive from Melbourne.

It's June 2004. School doesn't start until August. Rob is travelling six days a week for work and sleeping on the seventh, and apart from the awkward presence of the maid he hired – the norm for non-Thai-speaking expats – we are alone.

"Maybe this is an opportunity for Greta to take up something new, like swimming?" a new Australian friend I meet through an expat women's group suggests a month later as we sip chilled watermelon juice and I confide my struggle to find a singing teacher who speaks English.

Swimming? Swimming gives people earaches and colds. There will be no swimming, except briefly, in the shallows of the beach at Hua Hin in northern Thailand, where we go for our first ever family holiday in a foreign country when Jakob arrives from Perth for Christmas.

We can't afford the hotel fees at the popular tourist resorts on the island of Phuket, off the west coast of southern Thailand, so our driver Khun Manit drives us to Hua Hin, which is only two hours from Bangkok. Khun is the Thai word for Mr, Ms and Miss, and is the polite form. In return, Khun Manit and his wife Khun Lamai, who is our maid, call Rob "Sir" and me "Madam". I find this embarrassing, and the lack of privacy excruciating, but in Thailand this is essential to help expats like us navigate everything from shopping to bill-paying, as well as the crazy traffic. I draw the line at having them live in, but Khun Manit insists on being my constant companion when I go shopping – with mixed results, as I discover soon after our arrival when I am searching for a cork board for my office.

"This Coke, Madam," he smiles, as we stand in front of the soft drink aisle of our local Carre Four supermarket.

But when it comes to navigating our way around Thailand, Khun Manit, is an expert, and his expertise is always offered in the same way: "My idea is …"

On Jakob's first day in Thailand, it's Khun Manit's idea for us to visit the King's palace rather than go shopping, just as it's Khun Manit's idea for us to holiday in Hua Hin rather than the overpriced Phuket. "I think is better, Madam," he says, nodding and smiling as he bids us farewell before driving our car back to Bangkok for his own holiday.

Without the convenience of our car and driver, we are restricted to swimming and sunbathing at the nearby beach – the two things I can't do, as I can't expose my leg to the extreme heat – which is why the photo of cool rushing waterfalls on the front of a local tuk-tuk parked outside our hotel the next morning looks so alluring. For just 1000 baht (30 Australian dollars) the tuk-tuk driver can take us to the cool waterfall in a local National Park.

"This could be a world record for a journey in a tuk-tuk," Rob says, as 132 kilometres later, we bounce along the long road back to the hotel, hot and sweaty, shaking the grit from our hair and picking the insects from our teeth.

We are surprised when Rob's mobile rings. It's his mother.

"Are you all right?" she says, shouting across the miles.

"Tell her we should have gone by car, but we're fine," I mutter.

"Shh!" Rob says, holding up his hand.

"There's been a tsunami," he says, when he hangs up.

"What's a tsunami?" asks Greta.

We don't know – until we see the news. At Phuket, the beach suddenly disappeared, stranding boats and people. Minutes later, a giant tidal wave rushed to shore, destroying everything in its path – the worst natural disaster in Thailand's history with 5400 dead, including 2000 foreign tourists who could afford a holiday in Phuket.

When school resumes, the usual joyous and celebratory mood of students and teachers greeting each other for the new term is replaced by quiet grief for those who don't return.

The tragedy of the tsunami merely confirms my fears and suspicions about the perils of a beach holiday or any other sort of outdoor exertion in this now-threatening unknown land. The only safe exercise for anyone, especially Greta, is vocal exercise.

"I think she will sing opera," declares Sophie Tanapura, the teacher I finally find two months later, when she and Greta emerge from the music room after her first lesson.

Opera! My own heart sings. Sophie speaks English, French, Dutch and Thai – but she only teaches classical singing, not musical theatre. A soprano herself, with the support of her husband Khun Pakdee (the MC at the later concert at the Sukhothai Hotel), she has formed her own opera company from the best of the young sisters gathered through a public singing program in Bangkok. Unlike the renowned Bangkok Opera, which relies on imported soloists, the new Metropolitan Opera of Bangkok aims to be fully Thai – except for Greta and three other adult expat singers.

From then on, between drowning in homework, Greta spends Sundays with me, as we wind our way through the back streets of Lat Proa with our new driver with the unfortunate name of Khun Pong, for lessons at Sophie's grand art deco home, set amid tropical gardens and ponds across from the printing factory that funds her artistic ventures.

"We've got one! We've finally got one," Mum says, clapping her hands in glee, when we return to Melbourne on "home leave" during the following school term break and Greta sings in her newly minted soprano voice.

"Talent often skips a generation," Mum says, her green eyes firmly focused on me, and into my head pops the image of my old high school friend Gail playing the piano for the school talent quest when we are 16, while my friend Claire and I sing *Money* from the movie *Cabaret*, with me playing the male role, wearing a tuxedo from the op shop and a top hat Dad has made from cardboard. We won, and the next day a friend's mother asked "So what's your mother going to do about it?" It seemed a strange question. What could Mum possibly do?

Now I know, and I'm determined to do it for Greta, who has real TALENT.

"She's got to do what I couldn't," Mum says, tears pouring down her face.

After concert performances of excerpts from *Der Freischutz*, come rehearsals for a full production of *The Marriage of Figaro*, with Greta starring as Babarina, with a small aria of her own. Khun Pong listens in astonishment as Greta trills away in the front seat while I sit in the back basking in the golden light of this reflected glory. There's glory at school too, where she stars in all the musicals, and at the local Italian restaurant just a short drive from our place, where she regularly sings jazz standards with a trio of middle-aged Thai musicians.

I've seen all the movies about child stars who are pushed and end up with horrible lives. But the romance of the dream and the subconscious desire to present my mother with a better version of myself, with a talent she can understand, overrides my doubts. As long as Greta is still singing when she doesn't have to – in the car, in the shower, around the house, in the street and in the playground – I tell myself she's happy, although she talks to me in code in front of her friends, referring to the Metropolitan Opera of Bangkok as "the MOB", as she's embarrassed to be learning opera.

My new friend Marg, an Australian artist who's been living in Bangkok for 13 years, is less convinced. She listens patiently to my breathless accounts of Greta's achievements and my obsessive involvement, until one day when I describe how I made and illustrated a birthday card for a school friend of Greta's, whom I've never even met.

"Jane, why are you putting all your creative energy into making a card for a child you don't even know?" Marg says. "Why don't you do something for yourself?"

I blush and put the card away. Marg just doesn't get it. I enjoy making cards. Besides, I am doing something for myself. I'm working as an online journalism tutor for News Limited, with a rotating quota of 20 students from all over Australia and even Fiji, as well as writing for a Hong Kong-based hotel magazine where I get to eat at Thai hotel restaurants and write about it. But her comment leaves its sting, painful and aggravating.

Shortly afterwards, Marg shows me a book. "You might like to do this with me," she says. The book is *The Artist's Way, the Spiritual Path to Higher Creativity* by American author Julia Cameron: a 12-step program like Alcoholics Anonymous for people to recover their creativity. But instead of giving up something, they are reclaiming it. Perhaps I'll finally "write something" as my mother wants? Just nothing about her.

For the next six weeks I join Marg and three other expat friends to give Greta some space and reclaim some of my own. One of the first exercises is to admit and name your dream. "I'd like to paint totem poles in the Amazon," one of the other participants declares. Another wants to write a book. Another wants to dance.

I'm stuck. All my dreams have been for my children. I want to write something, but what and how? Over the years, I've tried to make sense of the complex and cryptic relationships that dominated my life by secretly transcribing my conversations with Mum and writing mini stories, or recounting them in furious emails to friends. They're just notes and dialogue – like plays. A thought occurs: I've already written one play – *The Triangle*, about Nanny visiting us in Mentone all those years ago, resulting in my mother's ban on writing about her. Perhaps I can write another? I take out my *Artists Way* journal and write, "I want to write plays."

Writing it down just might make it come true.

* * *

But first I have to deal with a bigger problem – growing bigger every day. The 36-degree daily heat of Bangkok is making my leg worse. Our maid Khun Lamai insists on showing me how to reduce the swelling by lying on the bed with my legs against the wall. We lie there together, our toes pointing to the ceiling while the blood drains to our heads, as I try to explain that even if I lie there forever, the swelling will never go down.

I'm glad to have the excuse of working from home in air-conditioned comfort, as my thick compression pantyhose makes me sweat profusely in the heat. The pantyhose was prescribed four years earlier in 2000 when I noticed swelling in my "good" left foot, too.

"If my left leg ends up like my right, I'll jump off a cliff," I told the physiotherapist at the lymphoedema clinic in Melbourne, who diagnosed mild lymphoedema.

"This leg will never end up like the other," she said. "Not if you wear a compression stocking."

It made sense. I'd worn a compression stocking on my big leg since my final operation when I was 22. It was awkward, especially as it bunched behind the knee and cut into the scar tissue. But it had kept the scars and swelling in check. The physio in Melbourne had also recommended a new lymphatic massage to reduce the swelling in both legs before measuring for compression pantyhose. Massage was the new treatment for lymphoedema, which was finally recognised after women developed it in their arms after the removal of lymph nodes during breast cancer surgery.

For two weeks, I had lain flat on my back in a small private hospital in East Melbourne, as with light upward strokes ("like stroking a cat") the therapist massaged both legs, working upwards from the lymph nodes under my armpits, behind the knees and in the groin, and finally towards the thoracic duct in my chest to clear the drainage paths. The internal scar tissue from my many surgeries was an obstacle, but it was worth a try.

Between these daily massages, to soften the tissue both legs were packed with chunky pieces of foam, known as "chocolate blocks". These were bandaged into place until I looked like a half-finished Egyptian mummy. Naturally, the therapist was impressed with my attitude.

"Do you mind talking to one of the other patients?" she asked one day.

Of course! I was so well adjusted. Soon, I found myself consoling Prue, who was being treated in the same hospital. Prue was a big woman in her 40s who had developed lymphoedema in her left leg when she was a teenager. Her leg was huge, and like Prue, it wept regularly – leaching clear fluid into the sheets at night from lymphatic overload. Prue confided how she'd recently met an old boyfriend who'd rejected her as a teenager because of her leg. "Are you still carrying that leg around?" he'd said with mocking contempt.

Talking to Prue was like confronting the future I might have had if my mother hadn't found Mr O'Brien and I hadn't undergone all those radical surgical reductions in my 20s. The big keloid scars made me vulnerable to cellulitis, a bacterial skin infection, but when I looked at Prue with her weeping leg and eyes, I was grateful. I had scars, but I also had mobility, and I didn't have to change the sheets every morning.

I was also grateful for this new massage treatment. Miraculously, after two weeks in hospital in Melbourne, and with the help of the new compression stocking, my puffy left foot was back to normal. Even more miraculous, my scarred and lumpy right leg had improved.

"It's even a bit smaller than your other leg," the therapist had said with satisfaction as she measured my calf. I couldn't believe it. From the knee down my calf muscles looked almost identical. As long as I wore compression stockings on both legs, they'd stay that way, she said, and she prescribed thicker compression pantyhose, which required Herculean strength to pull on, giving me spectacular biceps.

I was delighted. I bought sheer stockings to wear over the brown compression pantyhose and walked down the street, waiting for passers-by to declare me a symmetrical imposter. The only thing they stared at was my funny walk – a slight jerk of my right knee, from my final operation when I had to learn to walk again at age 22.

The massage treatment made it even funnier. Without the lifelong extra weight on my right side, I felt strangely unbalanced, as if I might fall or float away. A few months later, thanks to the scarred pathways and the simple act of being upright for most of the day, my big leg returned to its former pre-massage post-operative size. The therapist wasn't surprised. All patients required regular massage and bandaging for "maintenance", she said. I could learn to self-massage and self-bandage, or visit the therapist and hospital regularly to repeat the treatment. That was the life of people like Prue, and mine, too, if I wanted to maintain the results.

I chose not to. I didn't want to be a permanent patient like Prue. At the time, I was running my own freelance writing and cartooning businesses while working as the cadet counsellor and editorial training consultant for 120 staff at Leader Newspapers – a job that required me to be vertical. My leg didn't leach lymphatic fluid, nor did it weigh the equivalent of a small child like Prue's. The operations had given me a passable symmetry from the knee down. At work, I wore black opaque stockings over my compression pantyhose and the black mismatched Mary Jane shoes Mr Watt still made for me. I felt normal, even if others didn't always agree. When I'd left *The Age* in 1996 a colleague had confided with embarrassment that the male colleague who sat next to me had called me "clubfoot" behind my back. I was surprised and embarrassed – for him. Whatever he'd thought, my leg was normal enough for me. Until Bangkok.

In desperation, I decide to try the lymphatic massage again, travelling from Bangkok to Sydney for treatment at a special clinic at Mt Wilga Hospital. While the physio unblocked my lymphatic system, I planned to follow my *Artists Way* plan, unblocking my creativity and writing something of my own.

"Have you written the great Australian play yet?" Greta asks when I call from Sydney to see how she and Rob are faring back in Bangkok. I haven't. I'm too busy catching up on student marking, and too distracted by the doctor's depressing comment when she examines my big leg, with its square warty toes.

"If they had just got you some compression from the start, it wouldn't have got like this," she says, clicking her tongue.

I'm surprised by Mum's reaction when I call her from Mt Wilga with this news.

"You've got to remember there is no cure," she says, repeating it several times to ensure I do.

I travel back to Bangkok with my bandaged legs stuck in the exit aisle of the plane. Once again, the treatment only provides temporary relief before the swelling returns. Mum's right. There's no cure.

There's no cure for writer's block either. Instead of writing the Great Australian Play or Novel, I decide to write a letter to my father, setting him straight about my role as the messenger in his divorce from Mum all those years ago. I haven't heard from him since our last meeting. I know he's moved from Conneware, but I don't have his address or phone number. I haven't heard from Juliana much either since our move to Bangkok, apart from occasional emails, where I gush about life in Bangkok and she replies briefly and politely. The divide between her and Mum and the divide between Dad and me has once again created a gulf between us.

"He's a bit bewildered about why you haven't been in touch," she says, when I finally call her.

I'm bewildered that he's bewildered. In our brief reunions, he treated me like an acquaintance he might meet for a coffee and a catch-up occasionally: someone on whom he could download his life, be affirmed and move on. He seemed neither embarrassed nor remorseful about his relationship with Doris. It didn't seem to occur to him that he should be.

It's all very confusing, and leaves me with nowhere to go with my feeling that my mother, me, and my sister have been wronged – and that this wrong deserves to be acknowledged and atoned for, although I can't explain this to Juliana, who's very much on his side, and who once again feels like a stranger. Nor can I explain it to Dad. I procrastinate about writing to him, and write to Juliana instead, sending her a long email on her birthday, about Jakob's visit from Perth, and how we've all been sick, especially Rob, and how I am sick of the heat and lack of privacy – the price we have for having "help".

She writes back, telling about her life as a social worker for the Salvation Army and being "nonna" to her grandson. We begin emailing regularly, addressing each other as "Sis", as if we're the same person, and just as our mother compared us, we compare each other.

"Wow! You're a good communicator on email," she says in reply to my elongated emails. "That must be the journalist in you. I'm more direct. I would love to have more confidence in writing, but I'm afraid it's one of my blocks."

I'm annoyed that once again she blames her inability to write on the competition forced upon us as children – which her perfectly written emails seem to contradict.

"There's no secret to it. Just write whatever comes into your head," I lie – without admitting that writing to Dad is one of my blocks. Writing funny stories about Bangkok isn't.

"See, the difference between you and I is that I would have told them to fuck off," Juliana writes, when I tell her how the stall holders at the Thai markets call out "Have big size, Madam," as I stroll past – and in my mind I hear my mother's voice saying, "She told the judge to fuck off."

Because I can write, she can't. Because she can tell everyone to fuck off, I can't. As always, we are shadows of each other.

***

Nine months later, on 20 September, 2006 we wake to find there has been a coup. Military forces loyal to the King have rolled tanks into Bangkok streets and declared martial law while Prime Minister Thaksin is in New York for the UN General Assembly. There is no TV or radio and the school is closed. In some ways, this is no surprise. Thailand has a history of coups – 17 since 1932 – and earlier that year there were mass demonstrations against corruption in the government and tax avoidance by Thaksin's family. We reassure friends and family who send frantic emails that there are no tanks in Samakee Place, which is 30 kilometres from all the action in Bangkok.

The next day, it's announced on national television that military forces loyal to the King have taken control without resistance. The army reassures the public that martial law is temporary, asks for their cooperation and apologises for any inconvenience. The apology is clearly accepted, as before long photos appear all over the media of the grateful public presenting bouquets to the bored but cheerful soldiers, many of whom wear yellow cloth armbands to show their loyalty to the King. The deposed Prime Minister is still in New York, and is not allowed to return home.

That's the only time I felt sorry for him. After three years in Thailand, I am homesick. The constant travel has taken its toll on Rob, who was discharged from hospital the day before the coup after a worrying illness and extensive surgery. Greta is also suffering constant allergies due to the pollution. My job as a journalism trainer is being reduced and my future career is uncertain, and well, I am yearning for cooler climes, a normal family life that doesn't risk the health of us all, and for my independence.

While friends and family at home admit to being wide-eyed with envy at the fact that we have "servants", they can't imagine the complex domestic relationships borne out of the inequities in Thai society and the many challenges that result – even when we tell them. Apart from the discomfort I feel about this inegalitarian situation, everywhere I go I am observed – at home with Khun Lamai, and while being driven by Khun Pong, who is so anxious to please that he angles his rear vision mirror in the car so that he can see my face as I sit in the back seat. If I cross my arms, he takes it to mean that I am cold and lowers the air conditioner. If I frown, he takes it to mean I am angry – possibly with him. It pays to be careful about what I say and what I do, although once I sneakily take a photo of the back of his head and send it to friends with the words "My view of Thailand."

I want to drive myself in all senses of the word, so I am relieved and excited when it is arranged that we will finally go home to Melbourne for good the week before Christmas, and that Greta and I will return to Bangkok the following July so she can perform the role of Barbarina for the MOB's premiere of *The Marriage of Figaro*.

Ironically, *The Marriage of Figaro* is a play about revolution – but against the monarchy of the time, with the plot centred around the servants usurping the monarch's right to have the first night with any local bride.

The production is a coup of another sort: a collaboration with Sophie and Maestro Dante Mazzola of La Scala Theatre in Italy, and his student Yoko Takahashi, a young outstanding pianist repetiteur who works at Sophie's house with the cast and the Japanese Mixed Choir of Bangkok. "The rehearsals are in Japanese!" Greta says in dismay after the choir members shuffle in bowing and smiling and wearing white socks and Japanese sandals and the occasional kimono. Luckily, Yoko also speaks English and can translate.

After 10 months of rehearsal, in celebration of the King's 80th birthday, with herself in the lead role of Susanna and Yoko conducting a 28-piece local orchestra, Sophie successfully presents the first local production of one of Mozart's most complex comic operas at the Thailand Cultural Centre. The Thai singers look incongruous in their 18th century-style wigs and costumes, but their voices are strong and their enthusiasm even stronger. To perfect their stage craft, they even take ballet lessons from a French former prima ballerina who lives in Thailand.

To help the local audience, instead of the usual recitative, the story is occasionally stopped during the performance while a Thai narrator (a local soap-opera star), dressed as an 18th-century country servant, comes on stage and explains the action in Thai. But in all other ways it is as credible a production as any, made more credible by the patronage of the Austrian Embassy in Thailand and one of Thailand's many princesses, for whom the audience must wait to arrive before the show begins and to leave after it finishes.

It's both a relief and strange when we all return to Melbourne the next day and resume our life in Australia – although I am confident returning is the right decision. After all, a Thai fortune teller had assured me of this fact.

Although I'd always been a natural skeptic, I'd gone with my artist friend Marg the week before we left, just for fun.

The fortune teller, a young Thai woman whom we paid 1000 baht for predicting our future through Tarot cards, stared at me and frowned.

"Take hair back – better for you," she said, and self-consciously I pushed my bangs back from my forehead.

Slowly, she fanned out the cards and asked me to choose, laying out my choices in a pattern before regarding them.

"You are very confused," she said, frowning again. "You think too much."

True.

She pointed to another card. "New job for you – three months."

My heart leapt, until she said the job would be in a restaurant. A restaurant? I wanted to sit in a restaurant, not work in one.

"Will going back to Australia be good for our family?" I asked.

"Yes," she said. "You have children?"

"Two – a boy and girl. Will my son live in Melbourne?" I asked, hoping to predict Jakob's future as well as my own.

"Yes," she said, and pointed to the Emperor Card, which she said meant success. "He older," she said.

"Yes," I said. "Will my daughter be successful?"

She pointed to another card, a knight. "Yes, but with support of your husband."

I assumed she meant financial support, as with a job in a restaurant I was unlikely to be much help.

"Will my husband be happy in his job?"

"No, not happy for the first six months," she said. "But healthy."

"Will my health be okay?" After all, one reason for returning was to help my leg.

She pointed to another card – a man carrying sticks.

"Yes, but hard work. Be careful back and leg."

It was my turn to frown. I'd been so careful for the past three years: carefully observing the local cultural norms, carefully managing a complex household, carefully ensuring my daughter had every opportunity. I wasn't planning to be careful. I was planning to be free.

23

Boronia, 2008

My little purple Hyundai Getz and I hum along together as I chug down the Eastern Freeway on the way to our house in Boronia. After our three years in Bangkok, I'm enjoying my privacy and the freedom of driving again. It's a pity Mum isn't enjoying it too.

"This is ghastly. I feel terrible putting you out like this. This is awful," she says, over and over, as she sits beside me.

She's coming to stay with us while Walter has an operation in the city. For some reason, she and Walter assumed she could stay in the hospital too, like a parent sleeping beside a sick child.

"Don't worry," I assure her, when the hospital refuses, "You can have a little holiday with us."

Rob has fully recovered and is in Hong Kong working in a regional role, returning home every six weeks for two weeks – when Greta and I frantically clean-up for his home-coming inspection. Living in hotels has made him forget what a family home looks like. Jakob is teaching at the Perth university where he's been a student and Greta is struggling at her new school.

"If you're Taiwanese how come ya speak English?" the kids ask on Day One, demanding to know which football team she follows, which prompts me to look for another school.

I'm still working from home as online journalism tutor for News Ltd, though with fewer hours – so I'm also supplementing my income by reviewing Melbourne restaurants for the Hong Kong-based hotel magazine I'd freelanced for in Thailand (which makes the fortune teller right). But suburban life feels too quiet after life in Bangkok, so we are selling our house, which, during inspections, has to look like no one lives there.

"We'll manage," I assure Mum.

One of the reasons we've returned is to help Mum and Walter, who are frail and old.

In the years we were away, I rarely spent any time alone with Mum. Our reunions during our home leave were family affairs. On the rare occasions I visited alone, Walter was ever present.

These days, he has a new name: "Ping". It reminds me of the children's story about the duck who lives on a junk on the Yangtze River in China, who is smacked for returning to the boat late one night. But Walter seems quite pleased with it.

"I've never had a nickname before," he says "Even the grandchildren call me Grandpa, never Pa."

To reciprocate, he asked Mum what he should call her.

"Bubbalina," she said, which to me sounded like Barbarella, the sexy but compliant futuristic space pilot played by Jane Fonda in the 1960s movie of the same name.

Alone in Boronia without Ping, I'm hoping for a meaningful chat with my mother to illuminate the questions that have lingered since reuniting with my sister and my latest reunion and break up with my father. Will my mother agree that I was the messenger and the cause of her marriage break up?

But as we drive along, I change my mind.

First, she complains about the lack of leg room in my car. Then she complains about the headrest, which squashes her carefully constructed chignon. Then she complains about the "fumes" from the road – even though the windows are closed. By the time we arrive home, I have a headache.

"Stop complaining and just enjoy the fact that you're having a cooking holiday," I say, as I pour her a glass of the excellent Margaret River wine I've been saving for a friend.

"I'm being told," she says. "That's what happens when you're old. Everyone's always telling you off."

"I'm not telling you off, I'm just asking that you relax, for all our sakes," I plead.

"Well, I hate being a burden. See – you're getting all rattled at having to do all these extra meals and things," she says.

"It's not the meals; it's your constant complaining."

"Well, I hate being a burden."

"The only burden is the complaining!"

"Well, I'll shut up then," she says.

But she doesn't.

"That's what happens when you're old. People are constantly bossing you around," she mutters when I tell her to relax on the couch while I put on a video of Bryn Terfel in *The Marriage of Figaro.*

She downs her glass and offers it for a refill, declaring, "Look at all the trouble you're going to."

"I'd have to cook anyway, so it doesn't make any difference," I say, to which she replies, "I love bananas, don't you?" as she picks one up from the fruit bowl.

Bananas are one of the few things she loves. Mostly she hates – and loathes – everything, even chocolate ("It sticks in my throat!") and ice-cream in a cone. "I *loathe* them! Lick, lick, lick – like a dog!" she says, licking in exaggerated pantomime, when I offer her one for dessert.

"Grandma, you loathe a lot of things!" Greta says in amazement. She's 15 and a keen observer of our family dynamics.

"How did you put up with this when you were growing up?" she whispers after dinner, when Mum is on the phone complaining to Walter.

When she isn't complaining, she's asking questions. "What's that?" she says, as I season the meal the next night.

"Salt."

"I love salt," she says, and proves it by turning every meal into a snowy landscape.

It doesn't matter. She rarely eats anything anyway. Whenever we visit in Castlemaine we take her and Walter out to lunch, where she orders soup and cake, eating three spoonfuls of the soup before moving on to the cake. The remaining soup is passed to "Ping", who eats everything she doesn't.

Marooned at our place without Ping, she arranges the food carefully around the edge of her plate, and declares herself full, adding, "Any more vino?"

Any suggestion she may not need any more "vino" is met with raised eyebrows and a declaration that they always have three glasses every night – one before dinner, one during and one after – which she regards as a mark of civilisation, rather than alcoholism.

She even uses it to wash down her many tablets, which are always arranged carefully on a saucer for all to see.

"Would you like a glass of water for those?" I ask.

She looks at me witheringly. "I hate water! Never drink it! I hate it!"

"Not even to have your tablets with?"

"Never drink the stuff," she says, with regal contempt. I should know. Once when I visited her in hospital carrying a water bottle, she frowned and warned, "You know water is fattening?"

"What do you have them with then?" I ask, wondering if I should make her a coffee to help wash them down.

"Wine or nothing. I just chew them," she says, throwing down a handful of fish oil tablets and masticating loudly.

I understand completely. The wine is necessary to help alleviate the anxiety, which by the end of each day has escalated for all of us.

"It's been lovely to see you all. Thank you for everything" – she says a week later after I drive her to hospital so she can join Walter in the Red Cross car for the trip back to Castlemaine. "You'll be glad to see the back of me."

Sad, but true. She has been more than a burden: she's been a pain in the arse. I know my mother's behaviour is fuelled by anxiety and possibly the onset of dementia, but that doesn't diminish my disappointment. I have a lovely home, a lovely husband, lovely kids and a lovely job. I wanted her to see triumph not disaster.

As always, I write about the visit to make sense of it, detailing every complaint she made in one big complaint of my own – which I submit to the ABC Radio National program, *Life Matters*, which had previously broadcast a six-part series on our life in Thailand. The only detail I spare is how our mutual anxiety escalated when the hospital wouldn't discharge Walter until he had a bowel movement, and how the whole family waited on tenterhooks for him to birth the pooh that would liberate us all.

"And Jane Cafarella is still talking to her mother," the *Life Matters* presenter Richard Edy observes in undisguised bewilderment, when the broadcast ends.

"My God, you're a saint," Juliana says when I describe our week together. Since my return to Melbourne, we've banded together in mutual frustration in our efforts to help Mum and Walter, and their mutual efforts to complain and resist. I laugh when she tells me how she visited to see how they were getting on after Walter's operation, and Mum said, "No one is here for us. We'll manage. Always have and always will. You walk the last mile alone."

I sweat and stammer the following Sunday during my weekly call to Mum, fearing she or one of her many friends has heard the *Life Matters* broadcast. I'm relieved when she doesn't comment. She always boasted they only listened to ABC Classic FM and it seems it's true.

I don't tell Juliana about the broadcast. I'm too embarrassed. The only person I tell, apart from Rob, is Dad's sister Tess, hoping for absolution. Tess is the family truth teller, and haven't I told a family truth? Tess was my mother's confidant before she and Dad separated, just as she was everyone's.

"I'm a giant tit that everyone in the family sucks on," she always says.

Other times she's a "bucket of shit that everyone shits in", until finally she tells them she doesn't want their shit and begins to tell uncomfortable truths, until everyone gradually stops talking to her. "Blood is thicker than water," she recites bitterly, adding, "So is shit."

"You must really hate your mother," Tess says, when I show her a transcript of the broadcast.

I'm disappointed – and ashamed. The broadcast was cruel mockery and I'm sorry, but it's hurt and confusion, not hatred, that prompted it. My mother is a puzzle I have to solve. And Tess is just the person to help me.

We sit together on the long benches at her kitchen table in Brunswick a month later, Tess, her younger sister, Tina and me, like three matching canisters in various shades of grey and brown, as they tell me the story I've never heard – of how my parents met.

"He ran over her with a motorbike," Tess says, making small neat circles in her coffee with her teaspoon, stirring up the past.

"What!?"

"It was Tommy's bike. Frankie would borrow it while Tommy was at work," Tess explains. "Lorraine was walking across the road with some groceries and he knocked her over."

Uncle Tommy was Dad's big brother and the family was living in Mentone at the time.

"Frankie was mortified. He felt terribly guilty."

"Was she hurt?" I ask, alert as a meerkat.

Tina takes up the story: "She hurt her leg. I don't think it was broken, but she was laid up for several weeks."

I grin in delight and amazement. It makes perfect sense. He ran her over with a stolen motorbike and they spent the next 20 years colliding. No wonder my mother never told me this.

Frankie didn't have to go far to see how the patient was faring, Tess says.

"She lived across the road."

Across the road? So, they knew each other?

Tess shakes her head. "They'd never met. They thought it was pretty funny. We lived at 39 Florence Street, and Lorraine lived across the road at number 42."

Number 42? Nanny and Pa's place, the red brick Californian bungalow next to the State Savings Bank where my sister and I played as children.

"Lorraine was in a terrible state," Tess says.

"Because of her injuries?"

Tess shakes her head again. "He had matinee idol good looks."

"Like Tony Curtis?" I ask, recalling the photos of my father as a young man, with his dark corrugated hair and boyish smile.

"More like Paul Newman."

It doesn't matter which – both were the hottest movie stars of their day.

The accusations Nanny and Mum used to throw at each other over a glass of sherry suddenly make sense. "You were so charmed by him," Mum would accuse. "So were you," Nanny would sling back.

"They all were," Tess says, her chin tilting with pride.

The girls who appeared at the door asking for Dad's big sister Mary were all secretly hoping the handsome Frankie would be home too. They couldn't compete. The girl across the road whom Frankie had bowled over had bowled him over too.

"She was a lady. She wore those 50s dresses, with belts. And lots of chunky jewellery and red lipstick," Tina says, as she poured me another cup of coffee, sweet and hot, just like this story.

I smile, recalling Mum telling me how friends used to ask to borrow her clothes. She never let them. Even if she had, they would have been disappointed. It wasn't what she wore; it was how she wore it. There was something regal about her – which should have been a warning to Frankie.

Tess and Tina were besotted too. Tess was just 14 and Tina was eight. "I was a very lonely girl and Lorraine was very kind to me," Tess says.

But the most besotted was Lorraine, who fell head over heels in love with Frankie and the Cafarella household, a mecca for food, stories and music – for which they were famous. In 1950, when a train strike crippled the state, Radio 3DB sent a Rolls Royce around to collect them to perform on the radio as the "musical Italian family from Mentone".

I imagine my mother venturing across the road from No. 42 Florence Street, a mausoleum to her brother, the dead hero, into the vivid technicolour world of No. 39 – like Dorothy in *The Wizard of Oz*, who fell from the black-and-white world of Kansas into the colourful and fantastic Land of Oz. Motorbikes and music brought them together.

"And smoking," Tess says.

Smoking?

"Lorraine had one of those long cigarette holders. She'd say, 'Frank, bring me my *papieros*,' and he'd come running to light her cigarette."

Papieros was Polish for cigarette, although no one knew where my mother heard it, just that she liked the effect.

Neither family was impressed with this smoke-filled romance. To Nanny, the Germans and the Italians were one and the same – responsible for a war that killed her only son. Southern Italians were regarded with even more suspicion. In the 1920s, when Dad's grandfather and mother immigrated, they were regarded as the blacks of Europe, culturally and economically inferior. Mum's accusation that Dad wasn't "positioned enough" in Nanny's view comes back to me.

"Mum felt that Mrs Hill looked down on us," Tina says

Mrs Hill? After all these years Tess and Tina still refer to Nanny as Mrs Hill. That says it all.

Dad's father, Gaetano – "Old Cafarella" as Mum always called him – was the 13th child of a poor family born in Malfa on the tiny island of Salina, one of the seven Aeolian Islands off the coast of Sicily, Tess says. The young Gaetano had a "turned eye" and was deemed useless on the land – not that there was much of that. His father sent him to the local seminary to become a priest at the age of seven, from where he was eventually sent to the ancient Gibilmanna monastery in Palermo, where he was educated and forgotten. At 17, he ran away to Australia, where seven years later he married my grandmother, Angelina.

Indolent and arrogant, Gaetano worked when it suited him, preferring to swan around spouting politics. It was Angelina's father, Francesco Taranto – my father's namesake – who supported the family by working at a fruit stall at the Queen Victoria Market, and who saved enough money to buy their first home at 39 Florence Street, Mentone, a more affordable outer suburb.

"Nonno thought it was funny that the streets were named after Italian cities and towns," Tess says.

Like Lorraine, who lost her brother when she was 15, Frankie was 15 when his ally and beloved Nonno died.

When Frankie and Lorraine met on that fateful day in 1953, he was just 20 and had left school at 14. The parish priest pleaded with Gaetano: "Frankie is good at school, especially maths. He should stay on." But Gaetano sent Frankie to work and collected his wages, denying him the education that might have made him more of a prospect to the haughty Hill family across the road.

Frankie's parents were against the marriage too. Lorraine wasn't Catholic, and she was five years older.

"They thought she was too old," Tina says. "It was a big thing at the time."

Not big enough. Soon Frankie and Lorraine were engaged. But not for long.

"Frankie would break it off, and Lorraine would be at the door pleading and crying, and it would be back on again," Tess says.

I try to imagine my mother pleading for anything other than the bills to be paid, and my father saying anything other than, "So what do you want? A bloody medal?"

"The ring went back and forth 13 times. I even wore it for a while," Tess says.

There was a ring? Mum always said they couldn't afford one, or she'd lost it.

This vision of hot-blooded romance, compared to the cold war I witnessed as a child fascinates and astounds me. Whenever I asked my father what brought them together, he said "It was the red shorts," – the ones Mum wore for tennis. Even then, her signature colour was red. Like her, it demanded to be noticed. Whenever I asked Mum, she said she married my father for his "potential".

I am enthralled by this story of passion. That's amore! Just like the 1950s movie. In the decades of separation that followed my parents' divorce, I was absent from any sentimental reminiscing around the Cafarella family table about romantic meet-cutes and had never heard it. I wonder if Juliana knows it.

She doesn't.

"Dad told me they met at a theatre group," she says in astonishment when I tell her.

I understand why Mum never told me this. It was her folly – her pleading and crying at the door of No.39 that led to The Great Mistake. She will be embarrassed that I know. I think about the dress she had to take back, along with the dreams, when she learnt there'd be no church wedding – and how her youthful hopes for romance resulted in misery and betrayal. Hadn't we all done the same – fallen for someone who let us down?

It ended in tragedy, of course. All great love stories do. But in the tradition of virtue rewarded, the Cinderella love story, she finally met her handsome Prince in Walter, and lived happily ever after. Sort of.

* * *

A few months later, I am at home in my office working, when Mum calls, distressed. My cousin Joel, Doris's eldest son, had rung, pleading with her to reconcile with Doris, who'd been admitted to a nursing home with mild dementia. If they didn't reconcile soon, it would be too late.

"What should I do?" Mum asks.

"Don't do it," I reply, without hesitation. I know the plea hasn't come from Doris, who at that stage may not have even been able to recall who my mother was. It's a nice idea from my nice cousin, who'd lived in London for most of his life and hadn't witnessed the effect of the betrayal committed by my father and his mother. It's not an apology, or a plea for forgiveness. It's a plea for my mother to just forget it and reconcile so Doris can go to her grave with a clear conscience.

"If anyone needs sympathy it's you, not her," I say.

"You've hit the nail on the head," Mum says and she refuses my cousin's request.

Sometime after that, Doris dies. I don't register the year or the date. Nor do I hear from Juliana whether she or Dad attend the funeral. It doesn't matter. Doris has long since stopped being a person. She has become a symbol of my mother's betrayal; just as my cousins Pam and Pip have become mythical characters in the family story.

Three decades have passed since we last met. I wonder how Pam in particular, Doris's only daughter, felt about having my father in her life: whether she felt that her mother was justified in seizing the chance at happiness after a lonely widowhood, or whether she too felt betrayed.

Once I searched the Internet for her and found a brief interview on the ABC with an aged-care nurse with the same name. Nanny once said Pam was a nurse, but I wasn't sure this was the same person. I could have called the aged-care facility mentioned in the interview but I didn't. I'd led a public life as a journalist. Pam could have easily contacted me. But she didn't. The lines drawn so firmly all those years ago were difficult to cross for all of us.

24

I pick up the thick beige plastic hospital mug and place it on the tray table. "You won't feel a thing," I joke as I fill it with pink champagne to loosen my mother's lips and place my small unobtrusive silver tape recorder next to it, to catch what falls from them.

A year after Walter's operation, she is in the Epworth Hospital in Box Hill for a peripheral artery bypass – transplanting a vein to her leg to re-route the blood supply and alleviate the pain from the blockage caused by vascular disease. "Ping" is too old and frail to travel. It's my job to be there for her.

Blue and red bruises paint her right arm. The left lies limp from a recent stroke. The right leg, where they transplanted the vein is bandaged and elevated. Drugged to ease her pain, she's less anxious and strangely compliant, preferring to linger in the past rather than the present. The day before, she spoke sleepily about her childhood in Drouin, and it struck me that I should record it. I'd recorded Rob's father's stories before he died. I need to tease these stories out of my mother before she goes "to the cloud" as she and Ping call it. I hope she'll corroborate the love story Tess has told me.

To persuade her, I invoke her favourite mantra – "Tis but a short dance across the stage" – and begin by asking how she and my father first met.

She leans forward awkwardly for a mouthful of the champagne and sinks back on the pillow.

"He said he'd build a yacht and we'd sail away," she says, her words soft and slurred. I gasp. So, we'd both been seduced by a yacht – me by the Mirror yacht Dad and I were going to build when I was 16 and we were living in Heslop Street.

"Like the *True Love* in *High Society*?" I ask, recalling the boat Frank Sinatra and Grace Kelly sailed away on in the 1950s musical.

"Yes," she says, her eyes lighting up.

My heart jumps and I lean forward to catch the love story I know will follow.

"We used to go to Renmark to escape," she says.

Renmark? Renmark is an inland city in South Australia. You can't sail there.

With Dad?

"Dell and I."

Dell? She's gone further back than I wanted, back to when she was a student at the National Theatre Opera school and her cousin Dell was a student at the National Theatre Drama School. I go with her.

"Why were you escaping?"

"To get away from the Jew who was trying to make me marry him," she says.

I wince. Although she's used the term many times in the past, as a benign reference to the nameless boyfriend she refused to marry before she met my father, to my modern ear the reference feels like a racist slur.

"I didn't want to marry anyone," she says. "He was chasing me."

"You mustn't have had any love or lust for him," I say, hoping she'll confess to plenty of lust for my father Frankie, the handsome Italian.

"I never had any love or lust for any man," she says, disdainfully.

I frown, coddling the memory of the delicious love story Tess and Tina told me. Surely, she's lying.

"You must have had some for Dad because you went against everyone to marry him."

"I went against them because they were all getting at me," she says. "The town was getting at me. He lived across the road. I didn't have to travel anywhere – and they had music. I'm afraid the music got to me."

"But he was a good-looking man, wasn't he?" I say, hoping to trip her into a passionate confession.

She pauses, as if trying to recall his face. "He was very Italian looking."

"What's your ideal?" I say, feeling like the host on the television show *Perfect Match*.

"The Jew looked good," she says and I suppress a laugh. If she can't remember my father's youthful face, I doubt she can remember the face of the anonymous man she refused years earlier.

I top up her champagne and change tack, focusing on our days in Remo Street, hoping she'll recall how she and Dad managed to buy a house after going bankrupt in the milk bar business. A memory pops into my head – Julie carrying the milk bottle carrier Dad had welded – swinging it in ever-widening circles as we walked home from Cooney's milk bar. The four glass bottles with their silver foil seals rattled wildly. Then she let go.

"All the bottles flew out and smashed on the pavement," I say, laughing at the memory.

A cloud passes over her face.

"She was always a crank," she says. "Always going against everything. I was thinking the other day, why is she like that? There was nobody in our family like that. From the word go, from the first day of birth, she was a pill."

I stare at her in surprise. The demonising words that felt normal when I was a child feel outrageous now I am a mother myself.

"From the first day of birth?" I ask.

"She was. She wouldn't eat and wouldn't be cuddled."

"Did she cuddle Dad?" I ask, wondering if my sister preferred Dad, even then?

"Yes, all the time," Mum says. "She was a wild cat. A wild cat from beginning to end."

She's animated now. I've started something, and having started it, I dig for a deeper truth.

"You didn't like her much, did you?"

She is immediately affronted. "I DID like her. I loved her," she says. "I loved her little face. But I don't like her manner and her attitude. I don't like her attitude to life and people. I think it's tough and rough."

I think it's tough and rough too, but I see it as a defence, not a flaw. I think of all the times my mother asks, "Why is she like this?" so I ask her the same, hoping she might finally acknowledge her own part in it.

"She wants to disturb people," she says, fiery now. "She wants to be the show. She doesn't want the other people to get the show over her. She wants to own the show. She wants to be noted. As she didn't have any talents in anything … since she didn't have a talent, she'd be a nuisance."

Talent is how my mother always measures people. Still, I can't believe she's saying this about her own daughter.

"Nothing at all?"

"No. Not anything. What's her talent? She's an office person. That's not wonderful."

"She's a social worker," I say.

"She is not."

"She is. In the prison."

"Of course, in the prison," she says rolling her eyes. "That's just like her, to choose a prison to work in. Why couldn't she choose an office to be a social worker in?"

She sees my face and checks herself. "I don't mind her lack of talent. It's her perversity, I mind. Even as a toddler, she'd run away from me."

Lots of toddlers run away from their mothers as a test for independence. I make an oblique accusation of my own: that "perversity" may be a reaction to rejection. "Do you think she might have got the vibe?"

"No, because I'd cuddle her just as much, and she'd push me away," she says, and she repeats the familiar story from my childhood, about how Dad "took her into his arms from day one".

Is age masking the truth or unveiling it? Does she really feel that my sister wronged her from birth? Did she never feel anything for my father, for whom she'd sacrificed so much to marry? Did she really never love any man, as she claimed – even Walter, who is devoted to her?

Before I can ruminate further, she turns her attention to me.

"He didn't love you at all."

It should be a shock, but it isn't. I have decades of proof.

"I know that," I shrug.

"You do? You felt that did you?" she asks, with an interest that seems driven by curiosity rather than compassion.

"Of course."

* * *

I learn many important things in the weeks I visit my mother while she's recovering from that operation, and later when she's sent back suffering from a painful arterial ulcer. The eavesdropping silver tape recorder, forgotten under the pile of books and tissues on her tray table, becomes my witness to the conversations we share in a place familiar to us both, a hospital room-turned-confessional, although the drugs are no longer effective, and her pain and discomfort make her irritable and querulous.

"This is the worst hospital in the world," she says, when the nurses don't come quickly enough or refuse to give her unscheduled pain relief.

That year she turns 80, although we celebrated the previous year as I got the dates wrong. "It's my 79th, so don't bother," she said, when I rang her to tell her about the 80th birthday celebration lunch I'd organised at Celestine House, the bed and breakfast in

Guildford where we still stayed whenever we visited her and Walter in Castlemaine. We went ahead anyway, celebrating her un-80th that year and her real 80th the next.

She's in too much pain to care. She's worried about Walter, whom she fears is lonely and not coping. It doesn't help that he calls every day to tell her that he's lonely and not coping.

One afternoon, to distract her from her pain, I offer to turn on the television. She snorts with contempt. "I never watch television during the day."

That thought triggers another thought – about how she and Walter coincidentally watched the same television program the previous night, Mum from her hospital bed and Walter from their lounge room in Castlemaine. The program was about a woman suffering lymphedema in both legs.

"She just took no notice of it," Mum says. "I said to Walter, I hoped Jane would be like that, and say 'That's me, forget about it'."

My face burns. Forget about it? How can I forget what has to be managed every day? My teeth clench as she goes on and on about the wonderful woman on the television who's able to forget she has two big legs for which there's no cure.

"Now what did I say to you about your leg when you went to school," she asks leaning forward on her pillows. "See if you can remember."

And as if she's conjured up my child self, I dutifully reply: "Tell them you were born that way and nothing can be done about it."

She nods approvingly.

"There was nothing else to say," I say, snapping back to my adult self. "I had no information to explain it."

"Yes, but some children would have made a big thing of it and lain on the couch all day," she says.

Children accept things because they don't know any different, I say.

"It didn't stop the boys," she says, with a hint of pride, as if that alone is proof it was never a problem. Was this the reason she always said yes to me when it came to boys, and no to Juliana?

How can she know that such problems have to be managed every day – not just for the cameras during a television interview? To help her understand, I tell her what happened when I dared to forget it while walking from Kmart in Boronia to my car one day, wearing a short dress. As I walked, a woman in her 30s who was walking towards me, her eyes fixated on my leg, turned her head for a better look as she passed.

"It's rude to stare," I hissed at her.

The woman stopped and glared. "Shut up, ya fuckin' slut," she yelled, and shocked and shaken, I scrambled to the safety of my car.

Mum's eyes widen in horror. "It's dreadful, so dreadful," she says. "I understand now. I understand."

We sit with our mutual understanding, until she breaks the silence.

"Show me," she says.

What?

"I'm your mother. Show me."

"No," I say, and my 13-year-old self who had blushed as she'd checked my "development", finally asserts her right to personal privacy.

"All right," she says. "But I didn't cause it." She points to the heavens. "The man upstairs caused it."

I stare in astonishment. It never occurred to me to blame her or anyone. I was just born that way.

I smile and nod.

"I know."

25

The man upstairs has it in for me. "You've had a big day," the nurse says, handing me a glass of iced water as I stand in the doctor's office in East Melbourne.

I arrived for a suspected cyst on my right breast. Three hours later I'm leaving with a $1300 bill and a possible cancer diagnosis.

It's bad timing. Mum's back in the Epworth at Box Hill with an ulcerated leg. I visit her the day after I receive my diagnosis, forgetting about the small round white plaster on my bare upper arm, evidence of a blood test.

"What's that?" she says, so I tell her.

Two fat tears roll slowly down her cheeks.

"It's okay," I say. "It's only a tiny lump."

Thanks to the skill of the radiographer, the cancer was diagnosed early – Stage 1 – and the lumps are more like bumps – a tiny 3mm and 1mm – although the official diagnosis of Invasive Lobular Cancer a week later sounds scary.

"I'm not dead yet," I snort, after Rob confesses tearfully that he's "writing speeches in my head".

We've finally sold our house in Boronia and moved to an apartment in Richmond, to be closer to the city for when Greta goes to university. The week we move in, footy revellers trash the building and the stock market crashes, hurtling the world into the Global

Financial Crisis and threatening Rob's job. My diagnosis a few days later sends him hurtling down The Little Path of Gloom, which annoys me.

"If anyone's going to write speeches it's me," I say.

But that night, when he falls asleep and I am free from the need to reassure others, I think about what it might really mean. Greta is just 16. How can I leave her motherless (and stage motherless). Once again, she's starring in all the school musicals, while studying VCE solo performance in the hope of getting into the Melbourne Conservatorium to study classical voice. Jakob is 24 and teaching at the university in Perth where he was once a student. I blithely waved him off all those years ago, full of puffed-up pride that he'd been accepted into the most prestigious music course in the country. I've only seen him two or three times a year since. I hardly know him and now perhaps will never. And Rob and I have just embarked on an exciting new stage of our lives as city dwellers. How can I leave him now? I wake with a soggy pillow and a determination to survive.

"I know it will be all right in the end," I say, when I email the details of the diagnosis to Juliana. "I just wish I didn't have to go through the beginning and the middle."

My biggest fear is developing lymphoedema in my arm if the lymph glands are removed.

Her reply is brief: "Hi – reading this, taking it all in and digesting it. Will respond when I know what I am saying, love, me."

She rings a few days later. We have parallel lives. Dad's about to have a hip replacement. She's doing for him what I'm doing for Mum while coping with her own health problems. In the previous year, she's become so hoarse she can barely talk above a whisper. She's finally diagnosed with thyroid disease, which interferes with her diabetes and means that she, too, is in and out of hospital. We wish each other well, too consumed with our own problems to do anything more.

"Sorry again for the worst story I've never written," I tell the Education Age editor, when I fail my first deadline. The phone is running hot with calls from concerned friends and family who assume I'm dying.

"How are you?" a strange voice asks when I answer another call.

"Who is this?" I ask.

"It's Dad."

Dad! I haven't heard from him for five years – not since he blamed me for his divorce from Mum. Juliana must have told him about the cancer.

"How are you, love?" he says.

"Okay," I say, and I tell him the surgery dates.

He's about to go to hospital himself for his hip operation, and he tells me all about his pain.

"God bless you love," he says, when he's finished. I wish him well. I don't believe in God, and I'm too worried about my future to ask my father the questions still haunting me from my past.

"It was weird," I tell Juliana afterwards. "We really didn't have that much to say to each other."

I'm lucky. I keep my breast. The sentinel lymph nodes are removed but no further cancer is detected. No chemotherapy is required, just radiation and Tamoxafin for five years – the drug that stops the hormone-receptive cancer from growing.

The world is a marvellous place, and I'm still in it. Even the radiation therapy, which I attended daily for six weeks, is a breeze. I'm not tired, as everyone warned. I am a goddess, as the radiation turns my right boob into a golden orb.

"My right boob looks like it belongs to a 28-year-old tribal queen. My left boob looks like it belongs to a 82-year-old woman," I tell friends.

Rob gives me a new nickname: Miss Honey Dew. My surgeon offers to stitch up my left boob to match, but I've had enough of surgery.

So relieved am I that I'm not going to die from cancer, I write a story for *The Age* titled, Not Dead Yet, which ends with a poem about my proposal for Green Ribbon Day, to raise funds for all the people suffering from the common cold, for which there's still no cure.

I'm fine. It's everyone else who's suffering. In the year after her operation to replace the artery in her leg, Mum has been shunted from one hospital to another with ulcers and repeated infections.

That year, I attend the funeral of the mother of a dear friend. Not knowing anyone but my friend, I sit at the back and study the Order of Service, noting that the deceased, lying in a glossy pine coffin with gold handles, is only two days younger than my own mother. As the chapel fills with mourners murmuring their greetings, I notice the coffin is topped with a pair of slender gold-strapped dancing shoes, a tribute to her love of ballroom dancing. It reminds me of my mother's favourite expression about her short dance across the stage. Despite the many times I've cursed her, I feel a jolt at the prospect of her mortality, perhaps soon.

As I hear the affectionate eulogies from from the deceased's three grandchildren, my body buckles with uncontainable grief. Tears gush. My sobs are so loud several mourners turn their heads, gazing at me with sad consoling smiles. The woman next to me, who has maintained a dignified silence throughout the service, is shocked and disconcerted. "Did you know her well?" she whispers kindly.

"I never met her," I splutter, reaching for another tissue.

"Funerals bring out all the sadness in you," Tess says later when I confess my embarrassment.

From then on, I worry about how I'll cope when my own mother dies. Despite her callous talk when I interviewed her at the Epworth in Box Hill, her life and mine have been so entwined I fear her death as I fear my own. I need to be prepared, so I go to a counsellor – a middle-aged woman who'd found her counselling vocation after her young daughter died. Perfect. I begin by explaining my family relationships, which leaves her agog. I quit after four weeks, feeling no more prepared.

26

There are some things worse than death. Two months later, Mum is back in hospital to try to save her leg. The blood has stopped circulating and she's in excruciating pain. "Won't somebody help me?" she cries out in the night, and she begs to die.

An ambulance is bringing her back to the Epworth in Box Hill for tests to assess whether it's possible to do another arterial bypass in a final attempt to save the leg.

"I know you're having treatment," Walter says, "And I don't expect you to visit every day, but it would be nice if you could go for a short visit a couple of times a week." Of course.

Juliana is having an eye operation, a complication of diabetes, and is still struggling with the effect of thyroid disease, for which they've suggested radiation. Still smarting from a lifetime of rejection, she keeps in touch about Mum but doesn't get involved. She went to a clairvoyant who absolved her of all responsibility. After her thyroid stabilises, she and Macca plan to go on a cruise on the Rhine visiting the Christmas markets in Germany.

"I'm glad we will be away for Christmas and not have to keep anyone happy," she says.

I don't blame her. I confide my own conflicted feelings about our mother, and my struggles with a new writing project, paralysed by Mum's repeated comments about how she thought I'd write something someday.

"Funny isn't it, that you feel paralysed in writing and so do I because Mum makes me feel inferior to you," Juliana says. "We are both caught in the trap. We all tell lies in some way shape or form, so rather than get mad at Mum when she downgrades Dad and their life together, I ignore her. I don't want to buy into something neither of them have let go of. The difference between Mum and Dad as I see it, is Mum wants us to achieve for her and Dad wants us to be happy."

We are both caught in a trap, but in my view, Dad wants Dad to be happy. And what's wrong with wanting your children to achieve? I effuse about Greta's schedule and achievements, a repeat of her schedule in Bangkok, ignoring Juliana's frank question: "Is Greta stressed? Youth is so short and then we are responsible for everything."

Of course not. It's me who's stressed.

That afternoon Rob and I are there to meet Mum when she arrives at the Epworth in the Red Cross car from Castlemaine. Her leg is the colour of red globe grapes, bloated and dotted with yellow-crusted ulcerated craters, the skin dry and cracked like a drought landscape. She's alone in her hospital room the next morning when she receives the news that there's no hope: her leg will have to be amputated the following day.

The news hits us like a tsunami. Rob goes to hospital to be with her while I try to meet a work deadline, fielding calls from Walter, who calls me every few hours for news, comfort and to tell me he's done all the research and is confident that Mum can walk again with physiotherapy and a prosthesis, if the leg is amputated below the knee.

I'm less confident. Her diet of mostly wine and cake means she is thin and frail. Her left arm is as weak and floppy as a rag doll, due to a torn tendon and mild stroke, and she can barely feed herself let alone bear any weight on it. She's always spurned exercise, wickedly mocking Walter when, determinedly and methodically, he lies on the floor for his morning back exercises. But there's no point arguing about prosthetics now. I reassure them both, while failing to reassure myself that my mother can survive this, that we can all survive it.

Ever since my father lost his fingers, I've abhorred amputation; the notion that parts of you can be cut off and you can survive, incomplete. My mother's impending amputation feels like a metaphor for all the parts of our lives that have been cut off over the years, and which can't be put back together, despite all our mutual attempts at reunion. I once read that in ancient times, amputated limbs were buried so the owner and the limb could be reunited in the afterlife. Our family is like those limbs, buried, but still not whole.

I'm glad to focus on my work, grateful to be able to talk to Jakob, who's home for Christmas, and whose life in Perth has spared him the family dramas that dominate our lives.

"My Bubbalina," Walter sobs, when I take him to see Mum after the Red Cross car delivers him the next morning. I stay with him in the hospital all day, returning him after dinner to the hotel my stepsister booked for him. The spiral staircase in our new apartment makes it impossible for him to stay with us.

"Can you please buy a Christmas card and a Tattslotto ticket for Mum to give to me for Christmas? That's what she always gives me," he asks the next morning – a sad sign that he's unable to face the fact that everything is about to change.

He cries again when Jakob delivers him to the hospital later that afternoon. Mum's crying too. Nothing is right and no one can do anything to ease her pain. "This is the worst hospital I've ever been in," she says, but I know it's the worst situation she's ever been in.

I go home to finish the 12-page report I have to deliver by the next day. Rob takes Jakob and Greta to the concert where she's performing. I'll join them later after visiting Mum again before the operation the next morning.

As I set up the hospital tray table with books and toiletries, I babble on about the concert. She isn't listening.

"Have you heard from Juliana?" she says.

"No," I say and explain again that Juliana's on holiday and probably out of range anyway. I don't tell her that I tried to text her to tell her about amputation, but had no reply.

We talk about Christmas. We talk about Jakob. We talk about Greta, until finally she says in small voice. "I'm scared."

* * *

She's still asleep when I arrive at the hospital the following afternoon. Across the thin cotton blanket is a flat space above her knee where her leg should be. I know to expect it, but somehow it's unexpected. I begin to cry, loudly and uncontrollably.

She opens one eye.

"What are you crying for?" she asks in a small sleepy voice.

"Nothing," I blubber, wiping my eyes. "How are you?"

"Fine," she says, and she closes her eyes.

27

The notion of time takes on a new meaning after my cancer diagnosis and my mother's amputation. The *Artists Way* gave me permission to write but cancer gave me a real deadline. Galvanised into action, I enrol in a Council of Adult Education six-week evening playwriting course where I write four small plays.

My heart jackhammers as I read one aloud in class on fast-forward, fearing humiliation. Hadn't I failed at my first attempt at playwriting all those years ago with *The Triangle*, which led to the ban on writing about my mother, although this play isn't about my mother. It's titled *Presence* and is about a frustrated woman who's responsible for everything at Christmas – and who removes her presence.

"I've never heard anything read so fast," the tutor says in amazement. She's encouraging, observing wryly that I seem to be "always writing about disintegrating marriage". Two months later, the play is performed and published by Gemco Players, a community theatre group in the Dandenong Ranges, as part of its Little Gems series. As Rob and I sit in the audience together, I think of all the times I've sat in the audience clapping Mum and my children and I glow as the audience claps for me.

Mum is too distracted by pain to register when I tell her. Juliana has returned from the Christmas markets and been in touch.

"She's sounding positive about the future," Juliana reports.

Really? For the previous three weeks, Mum was in rehabilitation at Castlemaine, depressed, angry and in pain. They wrapped her raw stump in plastic film, leaving the flesh and bone exposed, like a leg of lamb in a butcher's window. All it needed was a sprig of rosemary. Walter was still convinced she might be able to wear a prosthesis, although this was unlikely, as she had no knee joint. She was too weak to do the exercises the physiotherapist had prescribed, and too distracted by pain to try on the soft pants and t-shirt I bought for her to make exercising easier. The pants were "too young" and the t-shirt showed her arms too much, she said. The nurses were mean and Walter wasn't supportive, she sobbed when I rang. "He's making all these lists. Why does he have to complicate everything? He took four pages of notes to the local doctor."

I knew she didn't mean it. I knew she was tired, sick, helpless and scared. As I helped her to the toilet, I saw that she'd cut her knickers around the top to stop the elastic from pinching. That's when she was wearing knickers. Most of the time she didn't bother. It was too painful to drag them over the raw stump. She forsook her pyjama bottoms, too, exposing her bald and infantile vulva, with its one remaining wisp of long grey hair. I placed a white towel over her lap to restore her dignity.

"I don't care," she said, when it slid off and I tried to replace it. It wasn't THAT hair she was worried about.

"I know what you can get me," she said as I rose to leave one day. "You know that stuff in the tube that I use to touch up my side bits on my hair? Can you get me two black ones?"

I didn't remind her that there were two tubes of Clairol hair touch-up dye sitting in her drawer from when she asked me the previous week.

When Walter called later that day to ask me to buy him "mid-tan shoe polish", I cut him off in exasperation.

"Does it really matter if you don't have polished shoes right now?" I asked.

Juliana is relaxed after her holiday, but I'm a pink drumming bunny, with batteries that never run out, going crazy with their demands and with the many freelance jobs I've taken on to pay for our new bigger mortgage, between running Greta to the rehearsals and singing lessons. When I pick up her from Box Hill to go to Doncaster Shopping Town, I take the wrong turn-off and get all flustered. I'm sure they've moved the freeway! All day I keep doing stupid things.

"What's wrong with you today?" she says, "You've been really strange."

"It's Tamoxifen," I reply.

Tamoxifen is the hormone-supressing drug, which has brought on instant menopause and sent my brain on holiday, as I tell Juliana in long chatty emails, although she rarely responds.

"Keep me posted about what's happening in your life too – otherwise I'll just go on and on about mine!" I write.

Eventually, she replies that she's having the same problem.

"I really think my thyroid is out to get me. Like you, it is making me stupid and flat."

She's moving to a new house in Bendigo, between going in and out of hospital to stabilise her diabetes and thyroid, for which the doctors have recommended radiation.

"We pulled up at the house on Saturday and I burst into tears sat in the car and would not get out. Real kid stuff. I am too flat to have the radiation at the moment and over the whole lot."

I know what she means. Five months after Mum's amputation, Jakob won a major music prize, ironically for a song about death. The prize included a special sculpture, with his name and the song title etched on a gold plaque on the front. After the ceremony at the Regent Theatre Ballroom, I was charged with taking the sculpture back to our apartment while he went to a party.

I arrived home with the cheque and the certificate but no sculpture, which remained lost despite desperate phone calls to the police and the taxi company.

Too mortified to tell Jakob in person, I emailed, telling him I was proud of him and asking him to remember all good things I'd ever done for him, as he would not be proud of me. It cost us $700 to have a replica award made. Not that he expected it, but it made me feel better.

"How will you feel if your cancer returns?" the surgeon asks when I refuse to take more Tamoxfin.

"I'll just have to take that chance," I say. I have more important things to think about. Like lamb shanks.

"I thought I'd just discuss the meal," Walter says when he calls to discuss my fortnightly visit. Mum has been discharged from rehab and he's caring for her at home with the help of a district nurse, although this is becoming increasingly difficult, as he's too frail and old himself to do the many transfers from bed to toilet. Riddled with guilt, every Friday fortnight I catch the train from Richmond to Castlemaine to help, bringing lunch.

"I thought I'd just bring some pies and cake," I reply. Pies and cake travel well.

Walter laughs his customary nervous laugh.

"We're a bit tired of pies," he says. "Don't bring anything elaborate but I thought some lamb shanks might be nice, perhaps braised, so the meat is falling off the bone. And if you could bring those little cakes Mum likes? And maybe some salad? I'll pay you of course."

"Don't be ridiculous!" I say, referring to the payment, not the request. It's the least I can do.

"Ah well, he's earned the right to be demanding," the lady in the homewares store smiles, as she wraps the large pot I buy to cook the lamb shanks in, when I explain that Walter is 87 and my mother's carer.

I nod, feeling both resentful and virtuous. I'm the only person who knows just how hard won that right has been. The many small strokes my mother has suffered since the amputation have affected her reason and on the rare occasions Walter is able to organise respite care, she feels banished and rejected.

As we'd stand together in the lift at Castlemaine Hospital one Friday morning, Walter leaning on his stick with one hand and carrying a plastic bag with Mum's clean washing in the other, and me with the usual offering of champagne and cake, he explodes in a flood of spluttering tears.

"What's wrong?" I ask.

"I know she doesn't mean it," he says. "She's irrational. But she told me I was trying to get rid of her," and he covers his face with his free hand and sobs.

After offloading the cake and champagne, I sit on the chair next to her bed and chastise her.

She turns to Walter accusingly. "I was only saying that to push you into saying something nice, because you never say anything nice. You never say you love me."

"I do. I say it all the time," he says, tearfully. "Every night, you say, 'I love my Ping,' and I say, 'I love my Bubbalina' – and other times too."

"No, you don't,' she says. "You're very cold. You just sit and don't talk."

He says he doesn't need pushing, and she only has to ask. She says she's just "a fiery person" and doesn't need criticising by him or me.

To my mother, my misplaced loyalty is yet another act of betrayal. "How would you like it, sitting here with one leg," she says turning her fury on me. "Your time will come," she tells me ominously. How would she like it if she was abused, despite trying to help, I say, pointing to Walter, who's almost blind in one eye and can hardly walk himself, he's so bent and crippled with arthritis.

"That's just the way I am. I can't help it. I don't mean to say horrible things," she says.

I can't help it either.

"You may only have a limited time left. Do you want to be remembered like this?" I scold, as Walter sits quietly weeping beside me.

She turns to me, astonished. "Like what? You make me out to be a horrible person. What have I done that's so terrible? I had no idea

I was such a terrible person to live with. Why are you attacking me? You're always on his side."

"Everyone's on your side, Mum," I say.

Later I wonder whether she's right. My anger is unfair and misplaced. Yet the interview I did with her at the Epworth in Box Hill before the amputation, where she claimed to never have loved any man, when she maligned my sister, for whom she seemed to have no compassion, made me wonder what sort of person she really was.

Since moving to Richmond, more and more I turn to my aunts Tess and Tina for answers, meeting them regularly at Trotters in Carlton. But like everyone, they have a question of their own: "Have you heard from Juliana?" Tess asks, as we peruse the menu we know by heart. I sigh. Juliana goes to ground whenever she is sick, overwhelmed or depressed and manages the relentless family inquisition by keeping her distance.

I'm glad not have heard from her. A month earlier, our cousin Angela, the youngest child of Dad's brother Uncle Tommy, died of ovarian cancer.

"What have you ever had to do with Angela?" Juliana said, when I told her I was thinking of going to Leongatha for the funeral.

Dad would be there, she explained, which meant she had "divided loyalties".

I was angry. It was okay for us to share our frustrations about Mum but not for me to assume I was part of the family. I went to the funeral anyway, enduring venomous stares from Juliana and an awkward conversation with my father, whom I hadn't seen for seven years.

The mystery of why no one has heard from Juliana leads Tess and Tina and me to talk of another mystery: how and why she ran away to Sydney at the age of 14.

"Mum was the only one who stood up for her at the court case in Wagga Wagga, and stopped her from being declared a Ward of the State and going to Winlaton (the home for wayward girls)," I say, as I sip my coffee, glad to find a moment of pride in my mother.

Tess's eyebrows shoot up and she draws herself up in that familiar way she has whenever she's outraged.

"She never said a bloody word. I was the only one who put their hand up."

What?

"She never said a BLOODY WORD," Tess repeats.

Neither did my father. Juliana was given over to Tess's care and she enrolled her in the local high school and paid for all her expenses. But Juliana played truant and was "endless trouble". The convent where she was finally sent to complete Form Four was my parents' last resort.

I can't believe it. "But Mum always said …"

Tess shakes her head. "She never said a bloody word."

There had been no one to contradict Mum's version of things over the years and it never occurred to me to question it. In all our talks about the past since our reunion, Juliana and I had never discussed what happened after she ran away at 14. It felt like a no-go area.

I'm beginning to feel I'm going crazy.

28

A year later, Mum is moved to the nursing home she always said she wasn't ready for, as Walter can no longer cope.

"Never in my wildest dreams did I imagine I'd end up like this," she says, looking around the sparse room.

We try to make it more homely. Walter brings the television from home, and I offer to bring photos and pot plants, but she refuses. It's not home; it's a waiting room before she goes where she really wants to go – "to the cloud".

"Here comes the good girl. Not like that other one," she cries when she sees me coming with champagne and cake.

"How are you?" I ask, although I know the answer.

"Awful. Just awful," she says. "I've had a dreadful life."

Her words cut me. If she's had a dreadful life then I've been a dreadful daughter, as wasn't it my job to make it all better? To make it all worthwhile?

"No, you haven't," I plead. "You've had 30 good years with Walter. Think of all the places you've been and the friends you've made. You've done art and had a lovely time."

For a moment, she's convinced. "I have, haven't I?" Then wide-eyed, she tells me about the debt collectors who came to the door when we were children and the secret money she earned from giving singing lessons; taking me back to the days when I sat at her knee as her confidant.

"Don't you ever tell your father about that," she says, leaning forward in her wheelchair conspiratorially.

No matter how many good years she's had with Walter, it's the still the years with Dad that haunt her, along with the bewildering thought that she's been abandoned – with "all the cuckoo people".

"People ask 'Where is your family? Why aren't they looking after you?' And I say, they're down in Melbourne, so there's nothing they can do."

I try to explain that even if she was in Melbourne, I don't have the skills to look after her.

"Yes, no one is expecting you to," she replies.

"Have you heard from Juliana?" she says, picking at her cake.

I have, but I keep quiet. Juliana is dealing with her own demons, one of which is Dad, who's also sick. To tell my mother we've been in touch will only inflame and distress her.

"I thought you might be friends one day," she says, with no thought of how difficult she made that.

"She only comes with Davina. Davina likes me. Davina makes her come," Mum says. It's true. The only way my sister can face Mum's accusing eyes is with her best friend Davina as a foil.

To distract her, I turn on the portable video player I've brought and we sit in the overheated room watching *Madam Butterfly*, and the operatic life to which she once aspired.

"Do you want me to turn it off so you can have a rest?" I ask, as her jaw slackens and her eyelids droop.

"What on earth are you talking about?" she demands, flinging her eyes open. "I wasn't asleep. I heard every word. I never sleep during the day. Never. Never have, never will."

I wish she'd give in to sleep, to age, to illness and to death. I wonder what I can say on her behalf when she finally succumbs or what she might say to me before she goes "to the cloud". In all our

234

time together, she's never mentioned what we went through when I was a child and a teenager as her sole confidant. Except once.

"I never said anything, even when I didn't approve," she told me on the phone once, describing how she wept as she and Shirley discussed my wedding menu.

I wish she had said something, anything. Just as I wish she'd say something now. I long for a few comforting words about what I'd meant to her then and now, the good girl, who perhaps hadn't been as good as she might have been. I long to know what leaving me means to her, and what I should say when she does. What music does she want? And who does she want to come to farewell her? I'm not being maudlin. I'm looking for guidance.

"How do you want to be remembered?" I ask, as she continues to resist sleep.

She opens one eye. "I don't care."

"But what do you want?"

She thinks for a minute, then looks me in the eye, half pleading, half challenging: "I'd like to be remembered as a good mother."

I stiffen. I look at her pale translucent skin, her thin stooped body, the greying hair that she still dyes with the help of a Clairol touch-up pen, the white towel slipping from her lap, exposing her knotty scarred stump. I know what I should say, what she wants me to say: "Yes, Mum, you were a great mother."

The good girl I used to be would have said it, but exhaustion, confusion and black fury has consumed all my loyalty and tenderness.

All these years I've heard about her pain, the pain of losing her brother, of being denied an education, of her thwarted singing career, of being stuck in a bad marriage with no money, ill health and two sick children, and of the pain caused by my sad and rejected sister and the husband and sister who betrayed her. In all those years, I was adrift, anchoring myself in other people's families with serial marriage – for better or worse. I want to scream, "It happened to me, too, you selfish old hag. I had no father, no sister, no aunts, uncles or cousins or grandparents. A good mother would understand that.

In her final years, shared with her daughter, a good mother might have something to say about what we'd both been through – together!"

But she doesn't say anything, so neither do I.

My blood is no longer worth bottling. It's boiling.

29

The blind is drawn and a lavender-scented candle burns on a small table nearby as Rob, Greta and I walk into my mother's room at the nursing home for the last time. She lies in bed, which is strangely elevated, covered in sheets and a long blanket. Her eyes are closed, and her mouth is slightly open. Beside her on her tray table is the dinner she hasn't eaten, a thick vegetable soup, beige like the plastic container it comes in.

I touch her hand. Her eyes flutter.

"It's me, Jane," I say softly. The smell of stale urine wafts toward me and I realise the scented candle is there to mask the smell of incontinence and decay.

Not knowing what else to do, I lean in so she can hear me and ask her if she wants some soup. She nods weakly and in a reversal of our roles from so long ago, feebly she swallows the teaspoonful I offer. It's not about sustenance: it's the last act of the will to live and an unspoken acknowledgement of the deep connection between us, of nurture and being nurtured, my final act of mothering my mother. Just as I've so often witnessed my mother performing, I too am performing the last rites of our relationship, hoping to release us both.

"I think your mother is nearing the end," the nurse had said when she called the day before. I didn't believe it. Six months earlier I'd waited with flowers, cake and lollies in the chapel at Box Hill Epworth, where Mum was being sent for palliative care, when I heard a familiar voice: "This is the worst hospital in the world," and I watched as she was carried regally like Cleopatra on a stretcher to the hospital room.

"She doesn't look as sick as you made out," the nurse at Epworth had observed wryly.

What did nurses know? The day before, when the nurse at Castlemaine rang with that final warning, I went to a movie with a neighbour. Later that night, the nurse rang again. "I think you should come now."

There is no escape for either of us now.

As the light fades and her breathing falls into a pattern of short gasps, Rob and I debate whether to stay or go and have dinner. We've driven from Richmond after work and are tired and hungry. After the death of Rob's father a decade before, his mother confided that, as he was wrenched from this world to the next, he let out a primal cry of pain. I don't want to witness such a final moment with my mother. I'd heard, too, that the dying sometimes preferred to be unobserved, sparing their loved ones from witnessing their final struggle. I suggest we go out for dinner and come back later. Appearances have always mattered to my mother; I will give her the dignity of privacy in her final hours.

"What do you want? I'll get it," Rob says as we sit together in a booth in the Cadillac Bar in Castlemaine, the only place in town that's open.

"Souvlaki," I say, and I concentrate on preventing the yoghurt dressing from dripping down my front.

"Nothing's changed," the nurse says when we call after we finish eating, so we drive on to the Cottage at Guildford where we're staying the night.

Twenty minutes later the nurse calls again. My mother died at 8.35pm. She was 83.

* * *

"Are you all right?" Juliana asks, when I call her the next morning to tell her our mother is dead. I was too tired to deal with my own emotions the previous night, let alone hers.

"Yes."

I was too numb to really know.

"Was it peaceful?" I asked the nurse after she rang us at Guildford with the news.

"Yes," she said. "I opened the window. I always think it's nice to let the soul fly free."

Perhaps it had, as at two o'clock that morning we were all woken by a magpie warbling – my mother's favourite bird – and the radio blaring.

"Where's the bloody radio?" Rob said, as we stumbled all around the cottage searching. In all our years staying there, we'd never used it. We found it on the lowest shelf in the bookshelf and silenced it.

Later Jakob told me that an hour before we'd called to tell him his grandmother was dead, he was playing at a gig where there was a clairvoyant. He asked for a reading, just for fun, and the clairvoyant told him she saw an old lady with a young man in an air force uniform. I hoped it meant that my mother was finally reunited with Joel, her brother and hero.

I don't tell Walter this. He is inconsolable. The weight he's carried in the past few years breaks like a dam. True to form, he has his lists. Now more than ever, it's important to follow correct procedure, including viewing the body, which is being prepared at the nearby Thompson's Funeral Home.

His insistence makes me wonder whether my sister should also be given the chance to say a final goodbye to our mother.

"I think you should see her," I say. "I can arrange it with the funeral director." Reluctantly, she agrees to go the next morning.

I wait for her at the Theatre Royal around the corner, with a glass of wine ready. They didn't sell brandy. It feels tragic and ironic that she finally agrees to see our mother when she's no longer capable of shaming her.

Fifteen minutes later she returns and reaches for the glass.

"I told her I disappointed her and she disappointed me," she says, and we both drink, dry-eyed, while I tell her the funeral plans.

There's so much to do. I choose my mother's final outfit: tailored black pants and the hot pink, fine-knit cardigan with the collar and gold buttons I gave her one birthday and which she'd hardly worn. I don't want to view the body. The only body I've seen is Rob's father's – curled up in the hospital bed like a fledging sparrow flung from its nest. But the day before the funeral, Walter insists that I accompany him to the viewing to take a photo.

"I think you'll be pleased," the funeral director says, as we enter the room. I watch as Walter staggers up to the coffin on his stick, and leans forward to deliver a final desperate kiss.

"She looks so beautiful, and so peaceful, thank you," he tells the beaming funeral director, and, exhausted from the effort, he slumps into the chair next to me.

It's my turn. I'm glad Walter is too deaf to hear my gasp. Her mouth is set in a grim line and the heavy make-up makes her look like a ghoulish shop manikin. I hold my breath and quickly take the photo, fearing her eyes, glued shut, might flick open like some horror movie. I smile at the funeral director, feigning gratitude, and leave, pushing the image from my mind. There's so much to do.

It seems appropriate that my mother is farewelled at a place called Agitation Hill, where in May 1853 the frustrated gold miners gathered to demand their rights, triggering a government inquiry into the unfair licensing system. A pretty sandstone Anglican Church now stands on the site.

"I'm only here for the social activities," Mum told the startled Anglican Minister at Maldon when they first moved there, but in Castlemaine in her later years, she began to hedge her bets, inviting the Anglican Minister regularly to her home to deliver personal communion in exchange for cake and coffee.

The funeral is "The Mum Show", I tell everyone. We'll all wear something red, her favourite colour. The coffin is decorated with red roses. Greta will sing *Ava Maria*, but only the Gounod version, Mum's favourite. Jakob will accompany her on the church organ and a parade of pictures will be projected to display her loving family – although I omit the photo of her lying bikini-clad with a burgundy tan on the beach at Lorne, and am surprised when Walter insists on including it.

Juliana isn't involved in these decisions. No one expects her to be. Mum was my problem. Dad is hers. I contact our aunts Tess and Tina, who are coming, but I don't contact him. He isn't welcome. I assume Juliana told him, and the rest of the family, whom I don't expect to see either. I keep her informed of the funeral arrangements by email. She declines to add any photos of her own to the slide show, but agrees to be included in some of mine.

It's the death notice, crafted by Walter, and the words "beloved grandmother of Melissa" – Juliana's daughter – that upsets her. "What had Mum ever had to do with Melissa?" she demands. It's too late to change it, so I email an apology, inviting her to publish her own.

There's no reply. Two days later I email another apology.

"If you're still coming, which I hope you are, would you like to say a few words? I'm fairly confused and upset myself, which is not made easier by everyone's demands," I write. And I tell her how Walter's daughter Jeanette asked that the funeral be held in the afternoon so she didn't have to get up so early, and how Walter asked me to bring my computer so he could email Jeanette the detailed map he drew of the church.

"He's hard work, isn't he?" the funeral director says after Walter asks to change the Order of Service for the third time.

To further win my sister over, I tell her how my friend Kaye still heard from her deceased mother occasionally and warned me to be open to the possibility, and how in the car on the way home from the funeral parlour, the CD from the musical *Gypsy* began to play with the song *You'll Never Get Away from Me* and how I was served at the supermarket by someone called Lorraine.

"Anyway, I hope you're okay," I sign off. "I'm a nice person, Juliana, and I care about you. I'm not Mum. Please don't run away and hide now."

I'm surprised and relieved to see her sitting in the congregation the next day, along with Tess and Tina and the neighbours of our childhood in Mulgrave, as I deliver the eulogy. With a small twist of the truth dial, I turn all the frustrations of the past years into quirks and endearments.

I don't look at Juliana, but I have a message for her: "In the past few years, whenever Mum was in the Epworth at Box Hill, I welcomed the chance to spend some time with her," I say. "In that time, she often said that while she didn't always understand us, she always loved both Juliana and me, and wanted the best for us." It's a lie, but I need to erase the truth as much for me as for Juliana.

She doesn't cry. Nor do I. Not until I mention Walter's devotion to our mother in her final years, when a hook unexpectedly gets caught in my throat.

As the mourners gather afterwards in the room behind the church for refreshments, I go over to see how he's coping. He wipes away a tear and tells me he's glad I broke down at the end of my speech and that he's very upset because Juliana said something rude about Mum to his family when they offered their condolences.

I feel sorry for him. How could he know what lay behind that comment? He must have been bewildered to see us both grinning instead of grieving while we cut the vanilla sponge cake that I ordered especially for the mourners afterward – with the words "Tis but a short dance across the stage," piped in chocolate icing across the top.

As I farewell the mourners outside the church, I see Juliana leaving.

"Come to Guildford and spend the night with me," I call. Rob is driving Jakob to the airport and Greta back to Richmond. I'm staying alone at the cottage that night to accompany Walter to the cremation in Bendigo the next day.

"Okay," she says, and she races home to Bendigo to get her diabetic supplies and pyjamas.

I don't know what prompts the invitation: fear of being alone with the ghost of my mother or the desire to share the evening with the one person with whom I shared a childhood?

The night is strangely balmy and we sit in front of the fire, sweating and drinking and talking about everything we remember and everything we don't.

"I hated you when we were kids," she says. "Mum used to say, 'Why can't you be like Jane?' When you were sick, she'd say, 'Don't go down there. Jane's sleeping.' I used to wish I could be sick, too. Then when I got diabetes, I thought, ooh I'm being punished."

A chill passes through me, despite the heat. I didn't know. "What about now?"

"It's different now. We're not competing."

The next morning, she leaves for work and I join Walter and the funeral director for the trip to the crematorium in Bendigo, squashed between them in the cabin of the hearse. It's raining and the slow thud of the windscreen wipers beats a funeral drum. The rain is nothing compared to Walter's tears. He sits with bowed head, weeping, the smell of unwashed clothes and dead skin mingling with our breath in the cloistered cabin.

I place my hand on his knee which is as thin as a broom handle, and we drive, with the rain and the tears, until we reach the crematorium, set in a pretty native garden with tall gum trees. I'm surprised when Walter says we need to choose an urn. I wonder why that task wasn't on one of his many lists. He chooses one in a dark grey metal with maple leaves etched on it. "Her last words to me were 'I adore you'," he confides, as we wait. I wish my mother had some last words for me.

Ten minutes later, a woman in a neat blue suit leads us to a room where my mother's mahogany coffin, stripped of its gold handles, rests on a tall stand. Uninvited and unannounced, the woman reads a passage from the Bible. As the coffin begins to glide into a curtained crevice in the wall, it occurs to me that my mother, wearing the hot pink cardigan with the gold buttons I chose for her and carrying the card Walter placed in the coffin like some sort of cosmic reference, is going to be incinerated.

Before I can digest this information, Walter lurches forward on his stick and places his trembling lips against the side of the coffin, moments before it disappears from view. The woman in the blue suit startles and glances at me, but I'm as inert as the body they've just committed to ashes.

On the way home, I pat Walter's knee again as he weeps quietly. The funeral director drives on unperturbed, his job and my mother's life complete.

My own eyes are dry. We had cremated Walter's wife, not my mother.

30

"If there was a thistle, your mother was sitting on it," Dad says, as he leans back in his chair and draws on his cigarette with his good hand. He turns the Redhead matchbox over and over with the pincer on his fingerless hand, while I marvel that he never considers who may have put the thistle there.

It's one year since my mother's death, and six years since our last reunion. He's sitting opposite me at Juliana's green and chrome kitchen table in Bendigo, ready to tell me all I need to know.

A month before, Juliana and I came to a place I never thought we'd reach. Walter was turning 90. I'd just returned from Singapore, where Rob had a new job and we'd escaped after Mum's death.

"You're welcome," I told Juliana when I invited her to the party that Greta and I were helping my stepsisters organise. But we both knew she wasn't. Walter was too angry and hurt that she hadn't visited Mum in her final months or contacted him after her death. So instead, I invited her for lunch the next day and listened as she told me all the things she was doing for traumatised clients in her job as a social worker, and for her daughter and grandson, all of which were challenging.

As she spoke, I felt a sense of wonder and pride. I thought of my mother's cruel words when I interviewed her at the Epworth. Why hadn't our mother felt this?

"I came away with a really good feeling about us, and a little sad, too, that Mum never bothered to find out who you really were," I wrote in an email the next day. "Any mother should have been proud to have you as a daughter. I'm proud to have you as a sister."

She replied within minutes, saying it "made her cry with acceptance and peace". "I always wanted to be accepted and am pleased we can feel good about us."

She told me she was proud of me too. It was my turn to cry. She didn't hate me after all. For the next few days, we continued to tell each other what our parents couldn't. I told her I wanted information from Dad. I needed to finally get his side of the story and discover for myself whether he was really the villain and "the Gigolo" my mother had labelled him.

Juliana offered to have us both over to her place for lunch – if he agreed. Tess warned me he might not. "He's got a strongly developed flight reaction," she said. Of course. Hadn't he fled every time my mother tried to confront him about the unpaid bills when I was a child?

I knew I had to be careful.

"How come you're suddenly interested in the villain?" he asked when I found the courage to call him to ask for an official interview.

"It was never as black and white as that," I said. "I need to know who you are in order to know myself."

"Well, when you find out, let me know," he joked.

I paused.

"Do you mind if I tape it?"

I had to get it right – the journalist's creed: accuracy, brevity, and clarity.

"No," he said. "I don't trust you."

"I just want the truth."

He laughed. "There's no such thing as the truth. There's only your truth and my truth."

And what was his truth? My mother was a whinger, a whiner, sitting on a thistle.

A week earlier, I'd received the same verdict from Doris's daughter, Pam. We met at Aunty Iris's funeral. Pam had gone searching for me, and I'd gone searching for her.

Loyalty had divided us. Death had freed us. We discovered we'd had parallel lives supporting our mothers.

"We could have helped each other," Pam said, as we toasted our warring parents with sherry, their favourite tipple – at a reunion lunch with Pip three months later. I was curious about what Doris had said about Mum over the years. Mum always had plenty to say about Doris.

"Mum used to say, 'As soon as Nipper comes, give her a sherry'," Pam said.

Was that all?

"She was a very positive person," Pam replied.

"How did Doris cope when the relationship with Dad ended?" I asked, keen for more.

"She just got on with it," Pam said.

Nor did Doris worry when Mum refused Joel's request to reconcile. "She just accepted she'd burned her bridges. She was a very positive person."

So, it seemed, was Pam. "There was always an attraction," she shrugged, when I asked for her version of why they'd got together.

Sitting at Juliana's kitchen table in Bendigo, facing my father, I feel a pang as I recall my cousin's implied criticism of my mother as someone who needed to be placated, and someone permanently discontented, sitting on a thistle, even if it was true.

But it's his truth I've come for, not mine, so I laugh companionably and feel in my pocket for the slim silver tape recorder I've hidden there – the same tape recorder I used to interview my mother at the Epworth all those years ago.

The betrayer is about to be betrayed. But first I need to win his trust, to anaesthetise him, like a spider with a fly, before I devour him. First, I need to show him I've been a victim too, and not the perpetrator as he cast me, delivering messages of divorce for my mother.

As my sister drinks brandy and pours tea, I tell him how difficult it was, being alone with my angry mother – confirming what he and my sister already believe.

"She was a bitch," Juliana says.

Feeling uncomfortably disloyal, I remind him of how my mother was always sick.

"She enjoyed the attention," my father says.

Not only was she a hypochondriac, she didn't keep her promises, he tells me matter-of-factly.

"I agreed for you to be raised Anglican, but she never took you. You may as well have been raised Catholic."

I am flushed as I remember the "body of Christ" – which I knew was just a wafer – distorting my mother's cheek after she returns, smelling of wine from Communion, to join Julie and me in the pew at St Augustine's Anglican Church in Mentone when I am a child.

Recalling my mother's illnesses reminds him of his own. "You don't get away with anything," he says, meaning his body is crumbling from the abuses of his youth, but which I choose to read differently.

"You think you do when you're young," he says. "You're invincible. I knew everything. I finally learned that I knew nothing then, and I've become wise to the fact that I know even less now."

How true. He alternates tea and cigarettes, enjoying the attention, anaesthetised enough for me to dare to ask the big question without risking him fleeing.

"How did you and Mum ever get together? You're so different," I say, smiling.

He smirks. "She lived across the road. It was easy."

So, no love story.

"Where there any good times?" I ask, fishing further. "Every relationship has one magic moment. What was yours?"

He doesn't hesitate.

"I was working for Eutectic, selling welding rods, and I had to go to Sydney for a while, and Mum came up on weekends sometimes. We went to a restaurant called the Beef Steak something and they had a piano accordion and violin and Mum started singing. It was fantastic. She was the absolute star," he said, his eyes shining. "She was happy."

I'm disappointed. The magic moment wasn't a moment of tender intimacy, it was a show and she was the star, just as she always wanted. It was a moment representing all the moments she missed out on after she married the hapless Frankie, her foolish Adonis, with the ring that went back 13 times, instead of having the courage to defy her parents and go to Covent Garden and become a real star.

I wonder what she really saw in the youthful Frankie, apart from his good looks, the music and his "potential"? I think about what drew me to Rik and kept me there, even when I should have left. It wasn't just our child that had kept us together, or that I had been painfully needy. It was his intellect and his story. Rik had had a troubled childhood, just like me. Was it the same for my mother? Had she fallen in love with my father's story, the story I felt entitled to know?

"Where were you born?" I ask, with a sudden urge to go back to the beginning.

"On the neighbour's couch," he says casually. "Mum and Dad were fighting and she ran next door to Marijuana's place and I was born on the couch later that night."

I'd heard this story once from Tess, but didn't want to believe my father had had such a sad and ignoble start in life – and who on earth was Marijuana?

"Italian for Mary Jane," he says. "She lived next door in North Melbourne. Dad never got over the stigma of it. I couldn't have a wee without being in the wrong. He used to kick me up the backside. I was a very skinny small child. He used to say I was weak."

"He was an orator," Dad says of his father, without realising he is also talking about himself. "He could swing a crowd. He could make a wedding reception laugh and cry at his will. He was big in the Italian community."

He pauses. "Ever heard of Arthur Calwell?"

Of course. And he tells me how Arthur Calwell, the Immigration Minister in the Chifley Government of the 1940s, who later became Leader of the Opposition in the 1960s, himself, used to sit in their front room at the Cafarella home at 6 Howard Street, North Melbourne, along with the Catholic Archbishop of Melbourne, Dr Daniel Mannix, talking to Gaetano, who was paesano (countryman), sponsoring new Italian immigrants.

"They were all top nobs," Dad says of the prestigious parlour visitors.

Old Cafarella's generosity didn't extend to Frankie. "I left school at 15 because Dad wouldn't pay the fees," he says, confirming what Tess has told me.

His first job was as an apprentice refrigerator mechanic. When a baker friend offered more money, his father sent him to work as an apprentice pastry chef instead.

"I loved it," he says and I think of all those Sunday mornings when I was a child and Dad made cakes and chocolate custard in commercial quantities, a habit from his pastry chef days.

He listed all the jobs he'd had since, too many to count. I can only recall welder, toolmaker, foreman, purchasing officer, salesman, and real estate agent working for AV Jennings when we moved to our new house – The Ashley, in Mulgrave, which was sold when I was 14.

"Why was the house in Redfern Crescent sold?" I ask.

"They found out about me living in Mulgrave. They found out I should have been informing them. And I decided that because I didn't want them on the title – I couldn't own it myself – I'd sell," he says.

They?

"The Bankruptcy Trustee."

So that explains why my mother thought he'd gone bankrupt twice.

Why did the bank allow an undischarged bankrupt to borrow money for a house?

"They were slack in those days," he says. "No one cared. These days, with computers, they can check how often you fart."

After the trustee caught up with him, he resolved to buy a home he could afford outright without the approval of the Trustee. This explained why our house in Heslop Street was such a dump.

With one confession in the bag, I search for another. What about George Perry, the man who'd persuaded him into the milk bar business and who'd been jailed for fraud? How did they meet?

He can't remember, only that Perry was an agent who encouraged those he thought could make go of a business to borrow money from the bank.

"He had a scam where he urged them to borrow more than they needed, so the business would be financed at double its value."

Dad managed two milk bars for Perry, one at 630 Bell Street, West Preston and one at 36 Rae Street, North Fitzroy. Perry took the takings and gave him a cheque for running the business. "It never bounced," he says, as if that's proof enough of Perry's honesty. Eventually, the scam was discovered and Perry was charged. Without Perry's weekly cheque, Dad couldn't afford to pay his suppliers and went broke.

"There was no understanding that I'd hoodwinked anybody," he says. "In the meantime, I had to give evidence in court. I was questioned by Galbally, which was quite an experience."

Galbally, the famous criminal defence lawyer?

"Yes. You think you can defend yourself in court. All you're allowed to say is yes or no to questions. They tried to make out that Perry and I were in cahoots. He defrauded for 250,000 pounds, which today would be worth 10 million."

Were you in cahoots?

"I was told to (ask the bank for more than the business was worth) by him, but I didn't do it."

"I was stupid," he shrugs. My mother was right; he's a fool.

But thanks to him Victorians today can buy a fresh loaf of bread on a Sunday, he says, and he tells me how he persuaded a local baker to challenge the big bakeries, such as Tip Top. Once, they'd chased him in their vans, like a scene from the Keystone Kops.

"I said 'Let me speak to someone' … Shortly after that they changed the law," he says. A law breaker and a lawmaker!

He's enjoying being the raconteur, the orator, so I ask him once again how he came to separate from Mum, hoping he'll confess an affair with Doris.

"I'm not blaming you. But you were the messenger," he says, repeating the accusation he'd levelled at me years earlier about delivering the divorce papers.

"I didn't know what was going on. So, I rang Doris, who'd been listening on the phone when Mum rang Nanny at night."

I nearly drop my tea cup. Doris was listening in on my mother's conversations with Nanny and was acting as an informant?

He keeps talking, as if eavesdropping on someone's telephone conversations is perfectly acceptable. (As acceptable as taping someone without their knowledge!)

"Doris and I had a coffee to talk about it and we hit it off," he says, smiling at the memory. "I was working at Hella at the time, and the annual ball was coming up, so I asked Doris. Hella is a company that makes lights," he explains.

"She said it wouldn't be appropriate, so she invited other family members to come with her. We had a great time," he says, picking up his cigarette.

I glance at Juliana who's been circling, pouring drinks and clearing plates. She doesn't react. Perhaps this isn't news to her?

"A great time?" I say. "So that's when you got together?"

He shakes his head. "We didn't get together until years after that."

Really? Calmly, though my face is burning, I tell him about the defining moment of my life; when my mother found the letter he wrote about taking the pins from Doris's hair and marrying the wrong sister.

He draws on his cigarette and shakes his head again. "I would have remembered a letter like that."

I almost laugh. What will he say next? "May God strike me dead!" as he so often said to my mother when he lied to her? But perhaps he's telling the truth? It's simply not important enough for him to remember.

"It's great to be talking like his," he says as we part, and tears form in his faded blue eyes.

I have no tears. I'm too focused on my treasure – the stellar moment with my mother at the Sydney restaurant, the news of his troubled relationship with his bullying father, his villainous ways, including tax avoidance and lying to the Bankruptcy Trustee and the scam the mysterious Perry lured him into. Later, when I research it, I find no reports of my father as a Sunday bread hero, but I do find the 1961 and 1962 newspaper reports of the case against George Thomas Perry, 42, of Bridge Road, Richmond, a licensed real estate agent and money lender specialising in the buying and selling of mixed businesses. Perry was charged with fraud and forgery involving 24,000 pounds – not 250,000. His brother Ronald, and two women who also purchased mixed businesses through Perry, were also charged and appeared as defendants. Dad also purchased two mixed business through Perry, but he was a witness not a defendant. A former lawyer himself, Rob offers his own view of what happened: "He did a deal – and gave information against Perry to get himself off the hook."

I'm not surprised. I'm more surprised about the other news – that Doris pimped on my mother, which then led to her relationship with my father.

"There was always an attraction," Pam had said. It was that betrayal that had led him to take the pins from Doris's hair – and to the Great Betrayal that divided our family. Mum was right: The Gigolo and the Monster.

A few days later, I write to Juliana, telling her I'm "more in balance" and that I hope it hasn't put her out of balance.

"You have your history and special understanding with Mum, just as I had with Dad," she replies.

I reassure her. "This may be the only time I talk to him like this, as I'm going back to Singapore on July 10."

And knowing I'm leaving her to the same fate she left me with Mum, I add, "No doubt he'll get more demanding as his health declines – just as Mum did. If you need me to help, I'll be there. Mostly for you."

Before I sign off, I offer a confession of my own. I tell her that Mum was wrong to use me as her confidant and messenger, but that I took advantage at the time. That's why my father's accusation hurt so much.

"So, I must take some responsibility," I say. "Not for the divorce – they laid the groundwork for that themselves – but my role in the whole saga. Looking back, I think I may have been an insufferable prig. I guess we all had our role to play."

Her reply reassures me. "You've had a huge weekend of versions of stories and reflection. Yes, we all had our role to play in it, however I think they determined whose side we would take."

***

My father offers no apology for the damage he did to our family. He doesn't believe in apologies, as he tells me a few months later. We're at Tess's and he's recounting a falling out with my sister some years back. They got over it, but it "changed the dynamic".

"If I punch your eye and I blacken your eye and I apologise two minutes later or a day later, you've still got a bloody black eye, and even if you accept my apology, you're wondering if somebody else is going to blacken your other eye," he says.

In December 2013, I return to Melbourne for his 80th birthday, held at Pharaoh-themed pub in Geelong. I have mixed feelings about attending, but I know it's important to Juliana, who arrives with her daughter and grandson, balloons, a card and 80 one-dollar coins – one for every year of his life. Tess and Tina are also there.

We've gathered to champion him, with no comment on the mess he's made of his life and ours.

Afterwards, I go back to Singapore as planned. The cleaving of my family has instilled a pattern. I am adept at moving on, attaching myself to new people and places, as is Rob, whose family moved around country Victoria for his father's work. But the Singapore humidity exacerbates my lymphoedema and causes recurrent cellulitis. Unable to leave the apartment much, and with no children to care for, I begin what I'd promised myself when I'd completed *The Artists Way* in Bangkok – and what my mother always wanted me to do – I write something, beginning with research for a full-length play about surrogacy. The compelling story of an expat woman I'd met in Bangkok who'd had three children without ever becoming pregnant, and of the surrogates and infertile couples I'd interviewed for Accent at *The Age* years ago had stayed with me. I wanted to know more.

Researching surrogates telling their stories on YouTube is at the top of my to-do list. Ringing Dad is at the bottom.

He's puzzled. One minute I'm courting The Villain; the next minute I'm ignoring him. I text to explain he's in my thoughts but I have mixed feelings. He rings the next day, but he doesn't understand time zones. I'm asleep and miss the call.

A few weeks later I'm packing my bag for yet another hospital visit when Rob comes in with a letter. I recognise my father's neat slanting writing.

"Dear Jane," he writes, "Our relationship is all on your terms, which is why I'm ending it," and he signs it "Your biological father."

I am shocked. I feel as if I've been served with divorce papers. Hurt and angry, I email Juliana asking her to explain to him that I'm already dealing with one demanding father in Walter, who's old, frail and lonely. I have no time or energy for this nonsense.

She doesn't reply. I'm not surprised. Divided loyalties.

I think of all the times I've reached out to my father over the years, and how he remained unreachable, treating me like a casual friend rather than a daughter. What had I done to precipitate this "divorce"? The more I think about it, the more I realise that the problem is not what I have done, but what I *haven't* done. In his mind, I haven't been there for him. The apple hasn't fallen far from the tree. Just as his relationship with me as a child was on *his* terms, he is now complaining that my relationship with him as an adult is on *my* terms. He is right, but what else did he expect? I am angry that he feels entitled to demand more of me, without ever acknowledging the effect of his actions – and inactions – on my life.

"You're like Dad – good with words," Juliana had said when we had reunited all those years ago. Words are all I have now.

It takes five goes but I finally write a letter of my own. For the first time, I tell him how I'd hoped he might have some empathy for a child born with many physical challenges and who was manipulated by an unhappy and proud mother; that I'd hoped he might have some humility and remorse for the outrageous blame he'd attributed to me – and for the havoc he'd wreaked on all our lives. Until then, he would remain merely my biological father.

"If you want to be anything more, let me know," I write.

I send it registered post. There's no reply, so I send it again. Still no reply. I send it again.

Finally, I ring Tess. "Did Dad get my letter?"

"Yes," she says. "Three times."

What did he say?

"Well, he wasn't happy."

Once, he calls me in the middle of the night, not understanding time differences. I answer groggily, but he hangs up.

And that's the end of our relationship. Neither of us either ever call each other again. In my mind he remains as he was on the last day we ever saw each other – his 80th birthday – wearing a gold paper conical birthday hat, with a red party whistle in his mouth and holding a sign that says "NOTHING", that Juliana had made as a joke, because that's what told her he wanted for his birthday.

"I can't come on Sunday, I'm seeing Dad for Father's Day," Juliana sometimes tells me as the years go by, unintentionally reminding me of what I've never had.

*　*　*

Three years later, I'm in London tagging along on a work trip with Rob so I can meet a producer about *e-baby*, my first full-length play – about surrogacy – when Walter decides to die. In the five years after my mother's death, he was careful with every movement, every step, and every mouthful, weighing himself regularly and recording whether "appetite" was up or down. All the skills he excelled in during his working life were employed for his own survival.

Finally, despite his efforts, he has a fall and is taken to hospital. Weak and tired, he has no more appetite for life. His customary nervous laugh is replaced by a quiet urgency when my stepsisters arrange for him to call me to say our final goodbye.

"I've always considered you a daughter," he says, his voice tremulous. "The same as Amanda and Jeanette. I've always been proud of you and your plays."

I'm taken aback by this message of love. Just like a daughter, I've often mocked his pedantic ways and how he drove us all crazy with his bizarre quests – the latest for a copy of the final edition of the *Malvern Gazette* in 1941, where his own father had worked as a journalist. (I could only find the second-last edition.) I've never called him Dad, and he never encouraged me to, but he's been the only person in my life who has acted in a fatherly way. I tell him I love him too, just like a daughter, and am surprised to find it's true.

31

The lounge room in Walter's unit in Castlemaine is uncharacteristically messy. Boxes, plastic bags and coat hangers are strewn across the floor. "It's chaos," Mum would have said, if she'd seen it. Greta and I, along with my stepsisters Amanda and Jeanette are clearing everything out, ready for it to be sold. It's taken three days, but we're nearly done.

"These are your mother's things," Amanda says, handing me a big brown paper bag.

I've waited five years to have the past restored to me. After my mother's death, Walter refused to part with anything. Her tablets remained on the kitchen bench, her makeup and combs and collection of costume jewellery remained in the bathroom. Her bras and knickers remained in the tallboy in the bedroom and her dark pink (almost red) dressing gown still hung on the back of the bedroom door. Everything in his possession, just as she had been

"He still talks to her every day," my stepsister Jeanette had explained. He wasn't ready to let go.

I felt powerless to argue at the time. He was their father, after all, and his grief was so much more palpable than mine, as he often told me.

"Just as well you didn't call me in the morning. I do my grieving then," he said if I called in the afternoon. Adding, "I suppose you miss her too?"

Did I? I didn't know what I missed, except the chance to make good and to reclaim something of my mother before she had become Mrs Walter Wilson.

I wait until I'm alone in our apartment in Richmond to go through the brown paper bag, pouring myself a glass of wine before emptying its contents on the bed. A collection of cards, letters and photos falls out, some wrapped in plastic bags brittle with age. I had rummaged through some of these as a teenager, looking for my birth certificate before I knew there were secrets. What will be familiar? What will be forgotten? What will be new?

I begin with the biggest card: hot pink with a picture of a red rose under a clear plastic overlay: "To my darling wife on Mother's Day." Familiar. My father gave this to my mother in Heslop Street when I was 15. He never usually gave her anything for Mother's Day, which is why I noticed.

I read the verse.

> *I may forget to say the things*
> *A loving husband should*
> *I may assume my tender thoughts*
> *Of you are understood*
> *But in your sweet and thoughtful way*
> *I'm certain that you know*
> *Your love and you mean more to me*
> *Than I could ever show.*
> HAPPY MOTHER'S DAY, DEAR

Underneath, he has written: *What more can be said?*

From Me, with "Me" underlined three times.

An apology of sorts from the man who didn't believe in apologies. New. Until then, I hadn't understood the importance of those words.

Had my mother considered the apology worthless – the damage already done – or had she kept it as proof of the recognition she hoped for?

I wish I knew.

I pick up a small white envelope, too small to belong to any of the cards. Two small drawings are tucked inside. One is a woman caricatured as a cow. The other is a man caricatured as a toad. I laugh, recognising them at once. The cow is Nanny. The toad is Dad's father, Old Cafarella. They're drawn in black biro in Dad's familiar style. New. I imagine my parents when they first met, bonding over this clever mockery of their tough and bullying parents. Things are getting interesting.

In a small clear plastic bag, sallow and opaque, is a small black cardboard box. I open it, hoping for the ring that had gone back 13 times. Inside is a stainless steel cigarette lighter with a boomerang and a kangaroo etched on the front. New. Tess said my parents bonded over smoking. Is this the lighter that ignited their passion, the one my father used to light my mother's *papieros*, the Polish word for cigarette she affected when they were courting? It looks like something you'd pick up at a service station. Nothing special. I flick it open. No flame.

A cache of small black-and-white photos with white borders spills from a fat open envelope. Familiar. Mum before Dad, sitting with friends, smiling and smoking. In another photo, my mother is in her 20s; her hair fashionably curled and shoulder length, wearing a tailored three-quarter-length coat, standing in the snow beside a tall serious-looking man with round glasses and a broad face. His straight hair is combed to the side and he wears a three-piece suit and knitted vest and scarf. They are day-trippers, not dressed for the snow. I flick the photos over, looking for dates. There's a name on the back in unfamiliar writing: BEN. The family must have liked Ben, as there's another photo of him with Nanny and Kerry, the young son Mum's brother never knew. Something tells me this is the nameless Jewish man my mother rejected. He looks kind and intelligent. I'm glad he finally has a name.

Another small rectangular blue box with Christmas motifs reveals a delicate perfume bottle with a red plastic top. Kaboka, Bourjois, Paris. Empty. I open it and sniff. Nothing. A gift card decorated with a lily of the valley, white with green leaves, falls from the box, with a message written in the coded language of lovers.

Seldom was a 'maid' so sweet.
Thanks for your help, my 'sweetest' Tweet.
Love from Tweet.

Was Tweet also Ben, or a fellow thespian in a show? It seems theatrical. How did my mother help him? I wish I had answers instead of questions.

I pour myself another glass of wine, picking up pieces of the past at random. An envelope catches my eye. The sender's address is pre-printed on the back in black cursive writing: 264 Union Road Balwyn. Doris. Inside are three small typed notes on Doris's personal letterhead, dated 3 July 1977 – two months after my wedding to Danny, when Mum is still living at Davies Street.

They are brutally curt.

Lorraine,

As mum is now very frail, and in her declining years, if you have any last vestiges of the duty you should feel toward her, you may come and collect her for drives and other outings, which she would enjoy.

However, I prefer not to have you in the flat. This is for two reasons, one of which is obvious, and the other is that I will not have you imposing on her at this stage.

Alternatively, if you, having some uncharacteristic change of heart, and should desire it, I will put Mum into a taxi with directions to your flat.

As you have never in your life done anything kind or generous for her, I feel that now, as you have absolutely no family obligations, you could show some consideration for your mother.

> *If you do not fall in with these arrangements, it will be obvious that you have no wish to see her again.*
> Doris

I feel a stab of pain for my mother.

She doesn't "fall in" as four days later, Doris writes again:

> *Apparently you are under a misapprehension about a number of things, and I suggest that we meet and talk things over in an endeavour to clear the air.*

Nor is the air cleared, as a few days later, there's another curt letter.

> *Mum goes into Donvale Private Hospital on Saturday 1st October for three weeks. Address – 1119 Doncaster Rd, Donvale*

Horribly familiar. I remember these letters and the anguish they caused, and the flower Mum picked and pressed into the family Bible after visiting Nanny in hospital.

The letters fit the puzzle perfectly. Mum as the victim, Doris as The Monster. How could she visit Nanny while Dad was living there? Impossible! She had no money to help Nanny either. She'd barely had enough money to support me. Yet the accusation that Mum had not been a good daughter points to another side of the story. Doris, widowed with three children, had been left with the responsibility of their parents in their old age. She may have been enviably "comfortable" but she was also burdened and lonely. With a pang, I realise I'd never heard a word of sympathy from my mother for Doris's plight at a young widow even before the Great Betrayal. But Doris's threat that Mum may not be allowed to see Nanny again if she didn't "fall in", felt childish and mean.

On the envelope, Mum had written, "RING IRIS". I hope Aunty Iris offered some consolation for the shock of finding that the sister who felt entitled to betray her also felt entitled to chastise her.

I lie on the bed, weary now with the pain of these remembrances. I pick up another envelope, addressed to Mrs F. A. Cafarella – Mum

– at Spray Street, Parkdale, sent from Centre Dandenong Road, Cheltenham. I recognise my sister's ant-like writing. The envelope is stamped July 1975, the year after our family is torn apart. Strange that my sister is writing to my mother then, when even to mention her name sends Mum into a rant about how she "chose HIM", my father. The letter thanks Mum for a birthday card. New. I am astonished. I had no idea that my sister and my mother were in touch then. Nor did I know that my sister was living in Cheltenham, just a few miles from where I worked at Standard News.

In another small plastic bag are dozens more Mother's Day and Christmas cards addressed to Mum and signed "Julie" as she was known then, with an X or a heart. *Have a lovely day. Enjoy your day. Thinking of you.* They must have been sent when Julie was still married to her first husband Peter, before she reverted to her full name. They offer no window to her life nor any questions or inquiries that might open a door to ours.

Another letter is addressed to Mum in Davies Street, Mentone, thanking her for her invitation to visit and promising to get back to her about dates. NEW! As far as I know, Mum didn't have any direct contact with Julie until their reunion in 1995, 21 years after the separation. I check the date. September 1975. I was travelling around the Victorian high country with my boyfriend Dale then – instead of studying to prepare for my end-of-year exams. Had my mother organised a secret visit with my sister while I was away? Why did she keep this from me? Is it really new or have I simply forgotten?

Another letter from my sister thanks Mum for the wedding gift. Familiar: the explosive pressure cooker my sister believed Mum had sent to kill her.

Yet another letter from Julie lists what her husband Peter gave her for her birthday. Yet another, written from hospital after Julie is diagnosed with diabetes, thanks Mum for the get-well card. Another thanks Mum for the gift of a silver cup after the birth of her daughter. Julie had to pick it up from the post office as it went to the wrong address.

I'd visited Julie in hospital after the birth of her daughter. Why didn't Mum visit with me, instead of posting a gift? Why did she continue to promote the great divide while conducting a private correspondence with my sister, albeit sporadically?

None of my sister's thank-yous invite further correspondence. The doctors are helpful, the birthday is enjoyable, and everyone enjoyed themselves. The message is clear: she is fine without us.

I sift quickly through the pile, searching for answers. Another letter from Julie is addressed to our house in Redfern Crescent. Why is my sister writing to us then, when she lives with us?

Thank you very much for parlour, and for being so good about it.

Parlour! The name the nuns give to visiting day at the Convent, where my sister spends her Fourth Form year after running away at 14. There are nearly 20 letters from the convent, all dated 1971. Familiar! I remember them arriving first at Alfred Street in Highett, and then at Heslop Street in Parkdale, but I don't recall the content.

I go downstairs to get the bottle of wine and pour myself the last glass. Over the next hour as I read the convent letters, I hear my sister's youthful voice, the voice lost to me when I was the "good girl" and Mum's "project" at Redfern Crescent and my sister was the wilful naughty girl.

Angry and confused, contrite and sad, the letters detail her trials and tribulations in the classroom and the laundry where she works; how the pimples on her back that are "killing her", how she punishes a mean girl by putting salt in her tea and is punished herself with dishwashing duty; her grateful thanks for the weekends home and for the "yummy food" Mum makes and how she sings one of Mum's big numbers – *Big Spender* – for "social committee" – the girls' recreation time – "and everyone enjoyed it".

Some letters include drawings copied from Peanuts cartoon books, with me as grumpy Sally, "angry when an assignment goes wrong". That figures. I'm still angry when an assignment goes wrong. Most are addressed to us collectively, "Mum, Dad and Jane".

Only one refers to me directly, describing how I slipped a gift into her bag during the visit. She calls me a "little sneak".

"It meant a real lot to me," she writes.

Another letter reveals the title of the book: *I Only Miss You Three Times a Day*.

It's my turn to say "I don't remember that." I wish I did.

On the back of the envelope, she writes: "Daughter. In case you forgot my name is Julie. You'd better not forget."

Sometimes the handwriting is unfamiliar and she confesses another girl wrote the letter for her, because she's supposed to WRITE REAL BIG LIKE THIS, but can't. Her minute writing seems to reflect her ever-diminishing self, although as the letters and the year wears on, she brightens.

> *Mother Anne's pleased me with me, I think. I hope. I'm really happy at the moment.*

A Christmas card from Sister Jerome congratulates her for "coming top", with another girl, in the Form Four Correspondence School exams with a total of 76 per cent, and for being awarded a Commonwealth Scholarship. Sister Jerome offers a final vote of confidence.

> *May you always be as good as you were with me in 1971.*

The next letter is soggy, and I realise I'm crying. My wine glass is empty but I'm overflowing. I begin to pack up the rest, when I notice another letter in my sister's tiny hand. It's addressed to Nana Cafarella. The sender's address is Buckley Street, Essendon. Strange. In the letter, Julie thanks Nana for sending her two dollars and tells her about her first day of school, where "Aunty Theresa", as Tess was known then, enrolled her. New! Why did Tess enrol my sister at school? Surely that was Mum's job? And why Essendon? We never lived there. In the same envelope there's another letter from my sister, dated March 11, 1971, written from the convent.

> *… I wrote to Tina and Teresa to apologise for my behaviour and told them not to come for a while because I'm not ready to appreciate them yet. After I get used of seeing you and not getting heated and upset I'll see them because I don't want to be awful to them when they've helped so much.*

So, it's true. When the magistrate asked, "Who will take responsibility for this child?" it was only Tess who put up her hand.

I lie on the bed thinking about all I have learned about the past 60 years in one afternoon. When the magistrate asked that fateful question, my mother didn't put up her hand. Instead, she chose to punish my sister, perhaps because she was angry, perhaps because she was at her wit's end.

Shame made her rewrite the truth for herself – and for me.

I lay on the bed, wondering how I would have felt at 14, running away – away from hurt and rejection and then finding myself punished and a prisoner; how I would have coped with a husband who fled instead of facing problems; and how I would have felt as a lonely widow with sole responsibility for three teenagers and my aged parents.

The room grows dark as I think about all that was lost due to hurt, envy and fear.

PART FOUR

Healing

32

Castlemaine, June 2018

"Don't look", Rob says, as with a stick, he gouges the insides of the gunmetal grey urn etched on the front with gold and rose gold maple leaves. Compacted grey dust – the combined ashes of my mother and Walter – fall onto the black soil.

My stepsisters Amanda and Jeanette stand by as Rob shakes what's left of our parents into the hole at the base of the *Remember Me* roses we've planted, one on each side of the path near the back step of the 152-year-old brick cottage we've bought in Castlemaine.

After more than 20 years of renting The Cottage at Celestine House in Guildford for our stays, we've bought a cottage of our own.

It's June 2018, the second anniversary of Walter's death. It's taken us that long to decide what to do with our parents' ashes, which have been stored at the local funeral home. Mum and Walter wanted them scattered at Lorne, their favourite holiday destination. But none of us fancy a long drive to Lorne. In our one unanimous act of rebellion, we are planting them in our new garden in our new home in Castlemaine, the place where I vowed to never return. But after 10 years of living in an apartments in Richmond and Singapore, we needed to put down roots. Castlemaine felt like home.

As Rob pats down the earth around the rose bushes with a spade, I recall the diary I found among my mother's possessions, where she wrote: *Had a day walking around Castlemaine on my own. Bliss!*

Guiltily, I wonder whether she would prefer her own separate final resting place, but it's too late. Rob has put half the ashes under one rose bush and the other half under the other.

Afterwards, we stand together while I read the poem I've written for the occasion, apologising for going against their wishes.

"If Dad and Lorraine had known you'd bought this house, I'm sure they would have preferred to be here," Jeanette says.

Greta isn't so sure. "What if they haunt us?" she says when I tell her later.

"I already feel haunted. What's the difference?" I say.

From my new kitchen window, I can see the spire of the Anglican Church on Agitation Hill where we farewelled them both.

Juliana isn't included in this rebellious act of sisterhood. She didn't come to Walter's funeral. Angry that she didn't visit Mum in her final years or contact him afterwards, he dropped her from his will. I felt guilty but powerless to argue against this decision. He'd been fatherly to me, but he wasn't my father; he was Amanda and Jeanette's. They didn't have a relationship with Juliana and never inquired about her. They were already sharing his modest estate with me, the daughter of the wife who had "come to the marriage with nothing".

Juliana doesn't ask if Mum left her anything, and I don't broach the subject. I'm too embarrassed. She'll get whatever Dad leaves, as she's his sole beneficiary, although the thought that she's been rejected again makes me guilty and sleepless. I vow to help her if she ever needs it.

"This is a surprise," she says, when I tell her we've bought the house in Castlemaine, 45 minutes from her place in Bendigo. After Rob and I moved to Singapore, the distance between us physically had been matched by emotional distance. She and Macca had visited us there once on their way to Europe, but for me the visit made the gulf wider: she was a tourist, going home to a busy job and family responsibilities; I was an expat, free from work and family responsibilities.

Now I'm finally putting down roots – fertilised by Mum and Walter.

"I've bought my mother's life," I joke, as Rob and I sit in Togs Cafe, where we'd so often sit with Mum and Walter.

"No, you haven't," he says, as we order soup and cake, and he reminds me that I have a loving family and that I'm a journalist and playwright.

Just as my mother wanted, I have "something of my own" – made possible by the enforced solitude of my six years in Singapore, where I had mostly stayed indoors to avoid the humidity and continuous bouts of cellulitis. In my first year there, I wrote my first full-length play, *e-baby*, about the relationship between an infertile woman and the surrogate she hires in the United States. It's not until now that I realise I've put Nellie, the surrogate, in the same position I was in – forced into an abortion – with the added complication of a religious dilemma. I produced the play myself – hiring a director, cast and crew – in Melbourne at Chapel Off Chapel in 2015 to critical acclaim. The following year, it was picked up by the Ensemble Theatre Company in Sydney, and by the Tasmanian Theatre Company in Hobart in 2017, where it was nominated for Best Production in the Tasmanian Theatre Awards, and Katie Robertson won Best Actress for her role as Nellie, the surrogate. The play also had a rehearsed reading at the So and So Arts Club in London in 2014 and was later produced in Cedarville, Ohio as a student production, and in London at Brockley Jack Theatre by Aequitas Theatre. It was published by Australian Plays and Stage Scripts in London and, bizarrely, translated into Turkish by an independent translator in Berlin. The companies that produced it were mostly small and independent and I barely survived the emotional and financial turmoil of it all, but it was a modest success.

My second full-length play, *d-baby*, was about donor conception, continuing the theme of displaced persons. My heroine, Dee, short for Deidre, was a donor-conceived teenager with no family – just a claustrophobic relationship with her domineering and needy mother, who was keeping a family secret. Like me, Dee was searching for herself and the truth. Until then, I hadn't realised I was writing about loss, without ever recognising my own.

* * *

Shortly after we plant Mum and Walter in our backyard, a big yellow envelope arrives from The Royal Children's Hospital in Melbourne, containing 45 pages of records dating from 1962 to 1975 from the FOI search I requested.

The request was inspired by the tattered little outpatient's appointment booklet from 1962 that I found among my mother's things – the only evidence of my time as an outpatient for petit mal.

I flick through the wad of pages of the FOI report eagerly. The doctor's notes, written in a tight cursive hand, have leeched into the paper, making the words grainy and hard to read. A magnifying glass reveals a pattern: "headaches", "very slow", "generally well", "has been well", "had a nasty turn".

A letter from Dr Coldbeck to my local GP reports: "… her reading has improved and her writing is almost normal" – meaning no mirror writing. It reads more like a school report than a medical report: "doing well at school", "school work very good", "school work excellent". There are only a few references to "leg swells in summer", which isn't surprising, as Dr Coldbeck was a neurologist, not a leg specialist.

At the end of the file, in a section marked "Correspondence", there's a typed letter from Mr O'Brien in 1975, seeking my medical records before my first leg operation when I'm 18.

Tucked behind it, is another letter from a Mr Reid to Dr Coldbeck, dated September 1964, when I'm eight years old. I squint trying to read the fuzzy type. I have no memory of a Mr Reid. It begins by thanking Dr Coldbeck for the opportunity to examine "this most interesting little girl".

"Apart from lymphoedema, this child appears to be suffering from a size 10 or 11 leg on a size eight child," Mr Reid writes.

Lymphoedema! In all my years growing up I never heard that word, not until I was 18, when Mr O'Brien diagnosed it. Until then it had no name, no cause and no treatment. It was just "my big leg" and I was "born that way". Yet here is evidence that it had been medically diagnosed at the age of eight by a mysterious Mr Reid, a specialist in East Melbourne.

Mr Reid recommends elastic bandaging in summer to ease the swelling, and a diuretic, and suggests a lymphangiogram may be done in future … the same procedure Mr O'Brien ordered before my first operation, where blue dye is injected into the lymphatic system to test its function.

I read the letter again in disbelief. They'd always known what it was and that bandaging, (known today as compression), would help, but the treatment was never implemented.

"You must be feeling gutted," Rob says when I show him.

Strangely, I'm not. I'm getting used to surprises. I'm sad and confused. Why did my mother let me believe there was no name and no treatment?

"Maybe she just didn't understand," a friend who is a nurse says. "When someone's dealing with the emotional impact of illness, the science can just become white noise."

My own frustrating experiences as a lymphoedema patient and the appalling ignorance amongst the medical community, means it's still often white noise. I imagine my mother trying to take in this strange ugly word and wondering how she'll pay for treatment. I wonder if Mr Reid told her what Mr O'Brien told me 10 years later: "There is no cure. It will never be normal." I don't believe anyone told her it was progressive.

"Maybe it was nothing?" I say to Greta, as I tried to understand why my mother never told me of this early diagnosis, or acted upon it.

"Mumma, anything that has to be managed isn't nothing," she says.

She is right. Managing it was my secret problem and gave me a secret identity. It was never part of my public identity, any more than being a breast cancer "survivor". As a child, I quickly learned society expected something more of the disabled and the deformed. (10 out of 10!) They had to prove something in order to appear deserving: climb a mountain, jump puddles, be a genius. Inspire us, comfort us, the world seemed to say, so that when you confront us, we can forgive you.

My mother taught me to ignore it so others would too, and by ignoring it, I avoided becoming a victim. I am immensely grateful to her for that. I doubt she really understood what the doctors said. I doubt she had the money to pursue it. She never doubted that I would cope. I was so well adjusted. It wasn't her fault. It was "the man upstairs". I was just born that way.

But I can't help wondering who I might have been if I wasn't.

33

April 16, 2019

The dusty brown paddocks and skeletal gum trees rush past in a blurry mist. I am driving to Bendigo to pick up some props for my latest show – crying. It's my mother's birthday. She would have been 91. She'd travelled this same road to Lansell Plaza every Monday to shop with Walter, as a perpetual passenger, inwardly railing at the rigidity of their life together and his clutching hold on her time.

Am I crying because I miss her? No. As Anchee Min, author of *The Crooked Seed* once said: "I don't have to miss China, because it never left my mind." We are cleaved still.

I am crying because she was disappointed with her life. When I reminded her of the gains, she could only cling to the losses.

"Oh well, let's change the subject," she always said, disappointed that I didn't understand. I did. It was just too painful to hear.

"I wish I'd been kinder," I say to Greta, as the birthday anniversary looms, and I recall the cache of cards with messages of love from Mum to me in Bangkok that I found in my own boxes of papers when we moved to Castlemaine.

"You can't keep on giving forever," Greta says.

I pull over, opposite Aldi. I think of calling Juliana, but don't. She's still too injured by our mother's rejection. I no longer blame my mother for this. Among all the realisations that have come to me since her death, is one that now seems obvious, and which is confirmed by a family friend who knew her when we lived at Redfern Crescent.

"She said she was pregnant when she got married. We just assumed she was. She and Frank were so mismatched," the friend tells me casually.

It all makes sense, the tumultuous courtship, the sudden marriage, Nanny's grim comments, "You made your bed, you lie in it." She is pregnant and then she isn't, as it's ectopic, implanted in the fallopian tube. She is trapped. A few months later she's pregnant again, and her monkey blood tries to destroy the child. The child is saved, but her husband's focus is the child, not what she has been through to birth it. At that moment, she hates him. At the moment, the man and the child are one and the same. She lets him claim the child.

That's my theory, anyway. Tess shakes her head in disbelief when I tell her. "We would have known."

Would they? Tess was 16 at the time. Tina was 10, unlikely to be privy to such shameful news. My father was her childhood hero and then a victim of his own folly, not a randy 22-year-old.

Of course, my father denied it when I put it to him at our final meeting the year after my mother's death. "Nothing like that," he said.

I hope she was. It's the only compassionate reason I can find for her rejection of my sister, although I never discussed this with Juliana. We are neighbours now – Juliana in Bendigo, and me in Castlemaine. But it's mostly holidays and birthdays that bring us together – or keep us a part, as Dad is her priority and my children are mine. Our lives are still siloed. She's never met my friends, except once briefly on my 50th birthday. I've never met hers, except Davina, once, briefly.

"I had hoped you could be friends one day," Mum often said, which always felt impossible. The connection we found after Mum's death fragments as I adjust to my new life back in Australia, while still battling recurrent episodes of cellulitis, and she copes with illness, the stress of work and Dad.

After lockdown we meet occasionally for coffee and lunch and thank each other for the lovely days, but we aren't intimate, and for me the lovely days feel strangely one-sided and empty. I'm still too wary of my mercurial unpredictable sister, who, despite our similarities, sees the world very differently.

"But I paid for them with my taxes," she says when I try to explain that the flowers in the public gardens are for everybody, not just her, and that picking them is against the law. She says she picks them for her clients – until a man from the council takes her photo and threatens to take her to court. "Get fucked," she tells him – and she continues to pick them.

In the car on the way home, I listen to Maria Callas, the voice closest to my mother's – imagining it's my mother singing to me and that I can ask her all the questions I never asked about how she did it.

"I thought you'd write something someday," she always said, which felt wistful and spiteful, knowing I was writing every day as a journalist.

I hope she'd be proud of the latest show I've written, which is opening in June at the Guildford Music Hall, around the corner from Celestine House, where we'd always stayed.

The show is *Uked! – The first play-along ukulele musical*, a sing-along, play-along love letter to the ukulele, which I took up while locked down in compulsory air-conditioning in Singapore. The humble ukulele, object of both ridicule and passion around the world, helped me reclaim my own musicality after years of promoting the musicality of my children.

Juliana had attended a few of Greta's shows over the years, but she'd never seen any of mine as they were mostly in other states or overseas. She seldom asks about them, and I don't tell her, feeling I'm forcing her interest and prising open old wounds about competing. Hadn't she told me often that she couldn't write, because "you're the writer," and because "Mum always compared me to you?"

Once, after we lunch together, she says in passing as I leave, "Your film's on soon, isn't it?" There seems no point explaining it's a play. She doesn't get it. Her only comment when I told her *e-baby* was to be produced in Missouri and Spain in 2019 by independent theatre companies – before Covid cancelled their plans – was, "Are you going to get paid for this?"

Yet after Mum's death she takes up singing and acting – going to lessons even when she is too hoarse to sing, and joins Bendigo Theatre Company, although I've never seen her perform. The one time she invites me it's cancelled due to Covid.

"Everyone else in our family is involved in the arts. I thought, why aren't I?" she says, when I ask what prompted her interest. She sounds like a child who's missed out. Soon it becomes her passion. Once, she was so excited about having the main role in a short play that in the rush to get ready she accidentally put Magic Silver White purple hair drops in her eyes instead of eye drops, turning them iridescent blue. She laughed about it but was heartbroken to miss the show and took months to recover.

Uked! is a musical. We both love musicals. When we first reunited, she bought us both tickets to *Beauty and the Beast* and *The Hunch Back of Notre Dame* – musicals about outcasts reclaimed. *Uked!* is about a lonely single woman who finds love and connection through the ukulele – another outcast reclaimed. I decide to invite her.

"No obligation," I say, keen to avoid further wounds.

I am surprised and glad when she comes. She can't sing-along. Her voice is too hoarse and painful. The next day she sends me a text, kindly ignoring all the technical disasters of the night.

"Your play was brilliant. Witty, funny, inclusive, sexy, and so true. You have a magical gift."

I'm touched.

After the show, I turn to the task I've been putting off after our move to Castlemaine – combining three former households into one: our apartment in Singapore, our apartment in Richmond and 10 years of documents, old books and toys from our storage unit in Scoresby. We had dumped all our personal documents in storage in the rush to move to Bangkok and hadn't looked at them since.

I wait until I've sifted and sold everything from both apartments before I bring the boxes from the storage unit to our little cottage in Castlemaine and begin sorting them on the dining room table.

Much of what's there I remember, including my baptism certificate from St Augustine's in Mentone, with my name spelled with two Fs instead of one, along school reports, photos, letters and reams of old stories from my days at *The Age*.

To the person I was 10 years earlier these documents would have meant nothing. Like the school essay, written when I was 15, about a dystopian future where the deformed and disabled are tried and put to death, and which I now recognise as a fine illustration of just how NOT very well adjusted I was. And the diary I wrote when I was 16 going on 17, where I echoed my mother's thoughts, expressions and judgements.

But it's the letter I wrote for her 48th birthday, when I was 18 that's the most revealing and disturbing. My scalp prickles as I read it.

When I was younger, Momma, you were my mother
The one who lit the fire in the old house at Remo St
That was warm
— not only because of that fire
But the fire within you
That glowed for your children and husband
The fire that kept you going above sickness, hardship and cruelty
You were the one
Who sang as you cleaned
That old house.

For five pages I list with poetic gratitude everything she's done for my sister and me, offering reassurance and absolution for my sister's rejection.

Although it is understandable, you grieve your loss, Momma, it is unforgiveable that you take the blame.

Remember that you know the truth of what happened and your relationship and Julie knows the truth, no matter what is said after that – the truth of the love that was and still is there remains.

I flinch to see how lost I was in my mother's story and identity. I had cleaved to her just as she cleaved to me – haunted now but possessed then.

I think of the time I complained to Tess that Juliana didn't support me and my work in the same way I supported hers.

"She can't. You were The Golden Child. She can never forgive the child who replaced her," Tess said.

The letter to my mother proves Tess right. I was the Golden Child, basking in the glory of my mother's approval and reflecting it right back to her. I made my own daughter the Golden Child too.

"A daughter is such a wonderful gift," a reader wrote, when Greta was born and I was writing the New Life Journal column for *The Age*. I agreed, and devoted my next column to the subject, writing that for the first time I understood why men identified with having a son, and about my fears for my daughter as she grew to womanhood in a man's world. I was immediately chastised by another reader, who urged me not to let my fears limit her. It was a warning that she was too precious.

My own mother wasn't kind – to others or herself. In raising my own children, I set out to be kind and joyous. Easter Bunny and Santa Clause in our house were playful poets, leaving clues in funny rhymes, and I determinedly shared all the books and musicals I loved.

But I was also anxious and too intensely devoted, especially to my daughter, unwittingly mirroring the claustrophobic relationship I had with my own mother.

When I realise what I've done, I call her. "I've got something very important to say to you and you're to listen and not say anything to make me feel better," I say. I apologise, and tell her it's okay for her to be angry: she doesn't have to console or forgive me – and I stop her when she says, "It's all right, Mumma."

"It's not," I say.

"Thanks, Mum," she says, after she hears me out.

We are close, but not in the same way as Mum and I were. Greta can tell me the truth.

"You were fun," she says when I ask her about our relationship. But our intense relationship meant that she didn't confide in her peers, she says. "I'd confide in you and we'd catastrophise together."

Nor would she have probably chosen to study opera, she says. As a teenager, she knew little about the pop music of her peers, which isolated her further – as did her unchildlike drive to be "productive".

"Greta is like her mother – a good manager," Juliana once observed, when I listed everything on her high school "to do" list

"My day was very productive," Greta says, when we call each other now, and we laugh.

She diverted from the path I set her on and made other choices that were better for her at the time, eventually coming back to music on her own terms.

My relationship with Jakob is different. The wall of framed certificates of his piano studies and awards in Boronia was an embarrassing testament to my maternal pride, but leaving home just before his 18th birthday to study in Perth saved him from the microscopic attention my daughter received. Sadly, it put emotional distance between us as well as physical distance, and which I'm only just reclaiming. I let him go too early and Greta too late.

In learning that I'm not a perfect mother, I learn to forgive my own mother, although I don't discuss these revelations with Juliana, just as I've never discussed the convent letters or anything I've discovered about the family and myself after our mother's death, fearing she will deny them or destroy them – or that they'll destroy her.

I'm surprised when she rings a few months after the ukulele show and confides her problems with Dad. He's 86 and living in a low-care aged care unit in Geelong. Naturally, he is slowly dismantling the kitchen and bathroom to "improve" it, while refusing to cooperate with the management and abusing everyone who tries to help him, including Juliana.

When he asks why he can't live with her, she tells him, "You piss yourself, you shit yourself and you stink. Nobody wants you."

He tells her she's cruel. "I wonder where I learned that," she says. Then she tells me how she made him a card and bought him a present for his birthday and took him out to lunch in the urine-soaked trousers he refused to change, enduring his rudeness to the staff and his loud exclamations that she was "Hitler" for not allowing him to smoke inside.

"That's not how I'll remember him," she says. "He was the only one who came to visit me in the convent."

I am silent. Should I tell her about the letters I found among Mum's papers after her death, with her own accounts of how we all visited her in the convent, including the letter telling us not to come because we deserved a weekend off?

I decide to tell her what I remember, not what I read, for fear she'll run away and this chance to connect more meaningfully will be lost.

"We visited you all the time," I say. "I remember the visitors' room. Mum felt so guilty she brought you roast chicken wrapped in foil and mice in blankets."

"I don't remember that."

I offer another memory. "You threw orange juice in my face one day when we visited you and had a picnic across the road at the beach."

Silence. Maybe she remembers that.

The conversation moves back to Dad. He told her he wanted to die, and she told him she prayed every night he would die peacefully in his sleep and put them both out of their misery.

I laugh. "When the time comes, I'll help you with the funeral," I say.

She pauses. "Dad doesn't want you at his funeral."

It's my turn to be silent. I haven't seen my father since he cut me off in 2013, shortly after his 80th birthday, and that's fine. I'm not sure I want to go to his funeral and hear the lies my sister and others might tell about him. But I want the choice, just as I gave her the choice to come to Mum's funeral.

We don't contact each other for a while after that. I'm angry at yet another ban on attending family funerals. Surely we've moved on since she told me I wasn't welcome at my cousin Angela's funeral in Leongatha. I feel confused and duplicitous, too, about withholding the convent letters I've found amongst Mum's papers. How will Juliana react if she reads them and sees that Dad, her hero, wasn't the only one who visited, and that he didn't pass on her sad and grateful letters to Nana Cafarella, thanking her for the dollar, "which came in useful".

For every memory I find, it seems she loses one. "I don't remember that," she says, whenever I talk about the past. My father and my aunt betrayed my mother, and now I'm betraying my mother and sister by uncovering the stories they are so ashamed of. But I can't help it. My own truth is so tangled up with theirs.

But as the months roll by, I miss her, so I invite her for high tea for her birthday. It's been so long since she's been to my house in Castlemaine she gets lost.

"We both love old things," she says, when she finally arrives, and sees we have furnished the house with French antiques, as the big Asian furniture we'd collected in Bangkok and Singapore didn't fit. My house is a dolls' house: pretty, but not always practical. Hers is a house of dolls, pink and white and black, dressed in old smocks and frocks and cardigans knitted by hands unknown, mostly from the op shop, where just as Mum did, she buys all her clothes. The dolls all have names. One represents the granddaughter she'll never have – as her daughter doesn't want more children. Some have things missing: eyes, hair, legs or arms.

"Why do you have all these broken dolls!" Tess exclaims when she visits. I know why. Juliana identifies with them, just as she identifies with the broken people she tries to help at work.

"They needed a home," Juliana tells Tess, although she's hurt at the comment. Still the dolls stare glassy-eyed and rouge-cheeked from their lacy pillows on all the beds and in cradles and prams against the walls of her 1930s style house, along with the rocking horse her husband Macca made for her.

The rocking horse, like the one I bought for Greta when she was small, is unspoken homage to our stays with Aunty Iris at the old house on the orchard at Williamsons Road, Doncaster, where we took turns to ride the big dappled grey rocking horse with the real horsehair mane. We both loved Aunty Iris and everything she represented.

We both loved Pip too, as we discovered when he died suddenly in 2016. He went to visit his brother Joel in London and developed a DVT. I wept when I read the email telling me he was gone, along with all the memories I'd shared with Pip, and Joel and Pam – and those I'd been surprised to find we hadn't.

"I don't remember that," Pip had said at our joyous 40-year reunion with Pam, helping himself to more garlic bread, when I reminded him of the day in Nanny's flat when Mum had found Dad's letter to Doris.

My feelings of fuzzy sentimentality, snap froze. "But you were there," I said.

"Was I?" he smiled. "I don't remember."

I puzzled over it afterwards. Perhaps Pip hadn't come when I'd called him that day? Perhaps he'd calmly finished his round of patience in the dining room while the storm that blew my mother and I away from our family raged next door in Nanny's flat like a trapped poltergeist? Perhaps it had never happened? But the play I wrote afterwards, based on the tape in my head which remained on continuous repeat, sprang from the wound inflicted when my mother found that letter from my father to Doris, as did the conversations that dominated our lives afterwards – along with the feeling that Pip had been my witness.

"I had a crush on Pip," I tell Juliana, when I tell her about his death.

"I did, too – except when he put a lizard in my bed,' she says.

Time has worn away the differences between us. We look like sisters. Our faces are both smooth and broad, despite our age, and we have a similar expression, although she's smaller and her hair is still brown while mine is various shades of grey.

"How come it's blue?" she asks when she first sees it.

"It's the light," I shrug.

Her nose, the one she chose, is still sculpted and as perfect as the noses of the dolls that surround her, but neither of us wear make-up and I no longer paint the fingernails I was once so proud of. Neither Juliana nor I are as glamorous as Mum was in her 60s. We haven't kept up appearances. The only thing we have in common with Mum is our mutual love of alcohol.

"Are you having a drink?" Juliana says, as she pours her usual brandy and diet Coke.

Brandy is the armour she still wears when she's with me.

"Shall we play some music?" I say after lunch. Usually, we play the songs Mum and Dad sang, with me trying to keep up on the ukulele: *Single Girl, Darling Go Home* and *Scarlet Ribbons*. This time I suggest it might be nice to play something she's learning at her singing lesson. She suggests *Funny Honey,* from *Chicago* the Musical, where Roxy sings about her husband's stupidity after he blows her cover when she murders her lover. I don't know the chords, so I find the YouTube video, and she sings along in a low voice, swaying to the music unselfconsciously in a way I never could.

I don't know whether it's the brandy or the naughty girls of Chicago that prompt it, but she begins to talk about her life in the convent. For "social committee" they had to sing a song about God, she says.

"I sang *Big Spender*. I lost privileges," she says, grinning.

Big Spender? I think of the letter from the convent where she tells another version of this story: "For social committee, I did *Big Spender*, and everyone enjoyed it."

Fascinated and guilty, I keep quiet about the letters again as she tells me how she escaped one night to ride the trams into St Kilda.

"Me and six other girls."

"How did you get out?"

"Hairpin," she says, as if I've failed to assume the obvious. They picked the locks and scaled the walls, riding the trams for free before the police picked them up.

"I got no privileges for a month, but it was worth it, just to get out."

For punishment, she had to polish the floors, and got her revenge by manoeuvring the machine over the habit of her jailer, Mother Anne, as she sat supervising.

"Nana Cafarella would write to me in Italian and send me holy pictures. That was the only thing that would settle me and bring me comfort," she says. "That and the visits from Dad." And once more she says he was the only person who visited her in the convent.

"Dad was my mother and my father. He taught me to take risks," she says, citing the time he took up archery and shot an apple off her head, which leaves me wide-eyed. She pauses. "He can speak five languages."

Really? I know he speaks Sicilian dialect, but I've never heard him speak any other languages. To prove it, she tells me how they attended a party where people had insulted them in Portuguese. "Dad answered in Portuguese and they shit (sic) themselves."

As if to fill me in on other things I may not know about my father, she says, "He made a gun. Didn't you know about that?" she says, when she sees my surprise.

How could I? It was the 70s and I was with Mum.

"Why did he make it? To shoot someone?"

"Because he can. That's what he does. He's always making things. The police confiscated it. They said it was really beautiful," she says, and I see in her eyes the same dazzled admiration I had for Mum as a child.

I don't know about her life with Dad, just as she doesn't know about my life with Mum, so in this brandy-fuelled atmosphere of confession, I ask her where they went when Dad took her with him as a child when he fled Mum's angry tongue.

"On surveillance, spying on Uncle Tony," she says with a grin.

On surveillance? I'd heard that Uncle Tony, Aunty Mary's husband, had a second family, but I hadn't believed it until Tess rang me after his funeral.

"That funeral was a fucking lie," Tess said, as she filled me in on the lurid details.

Now my sister is telling me she was recruited as Dad's spy.

"I loved it. Dad had connections," she says, pouring another brandy.

To whom?

"Bikie gangs, when he was driving taxis."

My father, who fled every conflict of his life, was involved with bikie gangs?

"If something happened, or someone needed something done, he'd say 'Let me speak to someone,' and it would be fixed," she says.

("Let me speak with someone!" Just like he'd told the bread companies who chased him in their vans!)

Mostly someone else did the dirty work for him, Juliana says. But once, he did it himself.

"He punched a man outside Aunty Connie's in Leongatha."

I'm astounded. My father is a fool, a dreamer, an artist, a crook, a tax avoider and, when it suits him, a liar; but the idea that he's also a violent gangster "fixer" seems incredible. It seems more believable when she tells me how he wriggled out of paying when they went shopping, challenging the shop assistants in cunning and charming ways.

The next day she sends me a text. "I spoke to Dad this morning and told him about our time together. He was very pleased for us."

"It's nice that he was pleased," I reply.

I'm not. The conversation throws me into a quandary, not about Dad but about Juliana. The contrite and lonely teenager I saw in the letters written from the convent was a crowing truant. And most disturbing of all, who was I? "The little sneak" as she'd called me when I snuck a gift into her bag when we visited her in the convent, was now an even bigger sneak, coaxing confessions from her without confessing that I know things: things she's conveniently forgotten.

When she leaves that day, I go to get petrol. The shop assistant's plump bare arm bears a tattoo of a pink rose on a green background. Tattooed above it, in fuzzy black script, are the words: "I forget whether I'm the evil sister or the good one."

"I know how you feel," I say as I pay.

I finally have the answers to my questions about our parents, but I've never fully examined how I feel about my sister. Over the years, she'd often told me how she hated me as a child, which made me angry and defensive. She never asks how I feel about her and until then I hadn't properly examined it. My focus was always my mother. But the more I found out about my mother, the more I discovered about my sister. It was Mum who'd asked her to bring a dog after Possum died, she tells me later. "I would never have done it otherwise. Then Walter came to the door and said they didn't want it." And once again, I am confronted by my former self who was so ready to believe ill of my sister.

When we reunited after 21 years, I was surprised at her constant talk of competing. I wasn't competing. I was relieved when she succeeded. It freed me to enjoy my own success. Why did she feel my success diminished her? It felt like a deliberate attempt to diminish me, in the same way Mum had diminished her by comparing her to me. Mum was right. She wanted to "own the show".

"You don't give anyone the opportunity," Greta says, when I complain that Juliana is always happy to talk about her work, but never ask about mine. "You interview everybody." And she points out how I fill the spaces, asking questions and cracking jokes, putting everyone at ease to address my own unease and deep need to be liked.

But combing through my own letters and papers has laid bare my own truth. I had enjoyed being the good girl, standing on the safe ground of my mother's approval at the expense of my sister. Juliana had good reason to hate me when we were children. And she has good reason to hate me now, for the story I thought was about Mum and me, but which I discovered was about us.

When we reunited, she had accused me of using words to mask the truth, but I was using them to find it, and her own words in the letters she wrote from the convent had led me to it, although I don't dare tell her. She's sick again, which is affecting her work, although she's reluctant to retire.

"I love my job," she says, even though the stress leaves her at war with her body. As she faces each battle, I invite her to lunch to offer support, not because she asks for it, she's too proud for that, but because hearing she's in trouble, troubles me.

"You've been through so much. Let me give you a hug," I say, as we stand in my doll's house after she recounts another stressful day. And she lets me. It's a strange but comforting feeling. We've never hugged, nor has Mum ever hugged us – at least not that I remember.

A few weeks later, I go to her place. "Did you bring the ukulele?" she asks after lunch, just as Mum had always asked, "Did you bring the guitar?" whenever Rob and I visited in Maldon.

It's the week before Christmas, so I play *Silent Night*, my favourite carol, and although her voice is weak and hoarse from thyroid problems, we sing it together in the tuneful voices of our childhood, blending in the way that only the voices of siblings can. Afterwards, we sing *Single Girl*, the lament of our mother, reaching for each other and the children that we were and the memories that we share.

The doorbell interrupts us. She hesitates. For the past few months, she's avoided company. As she gets up to answer it, I play on, not wanting to eavesdrop. Ten minutes later she returns with a gift a colleague has given her, adding that the colleague had asked about the music.

"I told her I'm having a lovely time with my sister," Juliana tells me, and she turns to the fridge for some more diet Coke.

A lovely time with her sister!

"Shall I get my ukulele?" she asks. She'd started learning a few years earlier, but the pain in her ring finger, swollen with suspected bone cancer, made it too difficult.

"You'll need to cut your nails. Short on your left hand and long on your right," I say, holding up my own left hand to demonstrate. I'm surprised when she promptly fetches the nail clippers and cuts them on the spot.

"Is your finger okay?" I say, noticing she hasn't polished the nail to cover the blackened parts as she usually did.

She holds it up. It's waxy and white but the nail is strong and clear. She refused the doctor's advice to have it amputated and treated it herself with ti-tree oil. The nail forms a crooked peak at the top. Just like mine. The irony of it, the sheer weirdness of it, strikes me. I hold up my own ring finger.

"What?" she asks.

"Look," I say. I point to the crooked nail line. "Just like yours."

"How did that happen?'

I stare at her. She doesn't know this story, just as she probably doesn't know any of the stories Mum told me when I was growing up, and which shaped my perceptions of my sister. I hesitate. I don't want to tell her, but she reads my face.

"Did I do that? How?"

"I don't want to tell you."

"Tell me."

"It's just Mum mythologising," I say. "I was in my pram, we were living at Croydon, and you were there … Do you know this story?"

She shakes her head, her eyes wide with anticipation. I repeat the story the way people repeat fairy tales: once upon a time … with all the familiar characters and phrases.

"... and Mum came in and there was blood all over my hand. She said you'd pulled the hood down on my hand. But I don't think you could have. You were only about two. I don't think it would have been possible. I must've got my fingers hooked around the hood of the pram. Croydon was bush then. Mum had to grab me and my finger and run cross the paddocks to the doctor with you hanging on to her skirts."

I show her the scar – a barely detectable line – and the tiny nick in the side near the nail where the top of the finger was sewn back.

"Oh," she says, and then with a hint of resignation: "I probably did. It would have been possible." And she tells me how a friend's son accidently slammed the door on his sister's fingers.

She shrugs it off, more interested in making music than raking through the past, so I teach her the C and F chords and she makes up a song about her dog. We sing the songs of our childhood again … which seem strangely prophetic: *The Sweetheart Tree*, about falling in love, *Lemon Tree*, about bitter betrayal, *Single Girl*, a mother's lament, and *Darling Go Home*, about a woman who betrays her darling with someone called Franz.

I think back to that day 47 years earlier when my mother and I left Doris's place in Union Road Balwyn forever in a taxi, the day I lost my whole family without anybody dying. It has taken 21 years to find my sister and 47 to find myself, and to understand what happened and why. My father's words ring in my ears: "There's no such thing as the truth. There's only your truth and my truth."

I have found my truth. My sister once told me she was writing hers. I hope so. My mother's words ring in my ears, too: "I had hoped you could be friends one day."

Perhaps we can? I wish she see could my sister and me, playing and singing the songs of our childhood, (although never as well as her, of course).

I wish I could tell her we are friends, and I am having a lovely time with my sister.

* * *

December 2021

On my 64th birthday, Juliana gave me my baby photo, enlarged and framed, and a one-page letter: *There's no one like a sister you haven't known all life long*, it began.

"How long did it take you to write that?" I asked, the tears pouring down my cheeks.

"Four hours," she laughed.

So, I told her about the book that had taken me nearly 40 years to write, and which I'd thought was about Mum but was really about us.

She listened and went to her filing cabinet and showed me what she'd been writing.

We laughed and we cried, and then we went to see *Frozen*, because it was about two sisters who were lost – and then found.

Epilogue

Memoir is by nature an interpretation in which others are unwillingly and unwittingly entangled.

In telling my story, I've been acutely aware of how it might affect those who were part of it – particularly my sister Juliana.

When we first read the book together aloud in February 2022, I wanted to know if it felt emotionally true to her. She said it did, nodding affirmingly as we read and stopped to discuss various incidents and anecdotes, including those where our memories differed.

I had worried that she would be uncomfortable about the revelations about her rebellious teenage years. But it wasn't her own past that worried her, it was mine.

"Aren't you embarrassed about putting all that sex stuff in?" she asked. She stared at me in amazement. "You were a root rat!"

I laughed. She had been shaped by Dad's Catholic prudery, just as I'd been shaped by Mum's relative liberalism.

She was even more astonished when I told her that the conversations and anecdotes in the book had been informed by everything I'd kept – diaries, notes, cards, conversations I'd jotted down to make sense of them, and 16 years of our emails I'd kept since we'd reunited in 1994.

While my policy was to keep and record everything, hers was to delete everything, following Dad's advice to destroy any evidence that might give someone the opportunity to pin something on you.

The day after we'd read the final chapter, she sent me a text, "Hi Sis, I feel great this morning – lighter and happier thanks to your dedication to write the book and commitment to research in keeping emails and not deleting anything, love you, your sister Juliana."

However, while it was healing it was also a shock. In her mind, our parents had separated when she was five-and-a-half and I was four-and-a-half, not 18 and 17. This is what she'd always told her husband and any friends who'd inquired. Confused, she asked to see the evidence.

We met at my place the following week. As she chattered over lunch before the big reveal, I felt sick. In the corner of the dining room was the big plastic K-Mart box containing all the documents – including all the letters she'd written from the convent as a lost and lonely teenager. I knew she'd find them confronting, as I had. I didn't realise how much.

As we read each letter of remorse and love, with her younger self thanking Mum for the delicious meals she'd cooked, and the clothes and cosmetics she'd bought for her, Juliana became more and more incredulous.

"Who wrote these?" she asked.

"You did," I said, pointing to her tiny writing and her signature, which had barely changed since.

"But I hated Mum," she said, tears pouring down her face.

"You were 14, scared and alone," I said. "And the nuns forced you to write to us every week, and vetted the letters."

The letters challenged her image of herself as the strong, defiant bad girl, and of Mum as a bitch and Dad as her hero.

"I feel as though I've lost my identity," she said as she left.

I worried about how she would recover, and that I'd put our relationship at risk.

The next morning, I sent her a text, apologising for upsetting her.

"You haven't upset me, I have upset myself by blocking the memories out," she wrote.

I was also challenged. While Mum had always accused Juliana of being "just like your father", through writing the book all the evidence pointed to the fact that the person who was "just like your father", was me.

I thought like Dad, I was erratic in my creativity like Dad, and I shared his love of words – and his cruel tongue. My sister was right: they got the wrong ones.

Throughout the next year, Juliana reread the book herself, and we shared many lunches and outings where we continued to find out more about each other and the things we shared, such as a love of yellow beans, a dislike of salmon and a love of old things.

The days together felt elongated and strange, as if we were in a time warp. We dubbed it our "bubble".

Once, while spending a rainy day in Castlemaine, we took refuge in a local op shop.

"Listen," I said, as we walked in.

The radio was playing Peter, Paul and Mary singing *Scarlet Ribbons*, which our parents used to sing together. The song is about a parent who hears their child praying for scarlet ribbons for her hair and is unable to get them for her, but miraculously finds them on the bed the next morning.

The next morning, Juliana sent me a text, "Thank you so much for our time-warp experience together yesterday … I spoke to Mum last night saying I forgive her. I love having a sister and enjoy the chats that show our similarities."

I had also forgiven Mum, recognising her as a woman of her time, frustrated and constrained by lack of education, money and support, and who had done her best. As I grow older myself, I realise that she was also battling the physical challenges of old age. I just wished she'd told me instead of always trying to keep up appearances.

Dad was another matter.

One of the similarities Juliana and I now shared was frustration with Dad, whom I hadn't seen since he divorced me in 2013, and who was struggling with health problems, too. He had flooded and dismantled the independent-living aged-care unit where he lived in Geelong, abused the staff and had been kicked out, owing money that he refused to pay.

Angry, he bought a house in Nathalia near Shepparton, sight unseen, where he abused anyone in the community who tried to help him. As usual, he dismantled the bathroom in order to improve it, but was too sick and tired to replace it.

He was 89 and suffering from vascular disease but refused to go to hospital for his gangrenous feet as he didn't want to leave his cat, his sole companion.

On the morning of July 25, 2022, Juliana rang me. Her voice was small and tight but matter of fact: "Dad passed away yesterday."

She was not sure when he died exactly, as he died at home alone – discovered by the health care worker who had arrived that morning to dress his feet.

She and her husband were heading to his house to collect the cat and to gather his personal effects. Rob and I offered to come too.

The death of an estranged parent is always difficult. In many ways, it represents the death of hope. So, it was for me. There was no hope now that my father would ever know how much I'd thought about him and sought to understand him. I wondered if he'd ever thought about me.

At the same time, I felt a strange disconnect. My sister's father had just died. My father had died a long time ago.

As Rob and I drove behind Juliana's car down a road as straight as an arrow, we talked about practical things and how Juliana would cope, especially as she wasn't well.

We arrived to find the police and the local ranger outside the house with the cat, a mangy spitfire, already in a cage, ready to go to the local vet.

The police had entered through back door of the house, which was open, which was just as well, as none of us had a key.

I had never been to this house, yet it felt familiar – the unmown lawns, the dirty dishes and half-eaten meals in the kitchen, the cement sheeting in the hallway, along with a new shower base for the bathroom he'd been too sick and frail to reconstruct, the cat and rat poo and unopened bills strewn all over the dirty carpet.

On a small table was a pile of red-bound books – a set of *Popular Mechanics* encyclopaedias published in 1968 – beside a small empty shoebox with the words 'dream big'. All my father's dreams were big, but few of them were realised.

Juliana reluctantly took the big baroque-style mirror that had belonged to our grandmother which she didn't like but Dad had wanted her to have.

I took the encyclopaedias in memory of all the projects my father started – and all those he never finished – and in memory of the brief time when we "dreamed big" together, when I was 15 and his eager apprentice, helping him renovate our run-down house in Parkdale (also never finished.)

Later that day I wrote a sad but truthful note on Facebook to tell friends about his death, mainly because I didn't want anyone to make assumptions about our relationship. It was a terrible loss but not in the way they might have imagined.

If my father had died two years earlier, Juliana would have been handling his funeral alone. I would not have been invited. I wouldn't have felt comfortable attending anyway, other than from curiosity about what other people might have said about him. I would, however, have fulfilled my mother's wish, which was to "dance on his grave". Instead, we organised his funeral together.

Juliana kept her cool. I lost mine. As I listened to the eulogies from other family members, I wept for my father and for all the things I never knew about him, including that he loved the film *Seven Brides for Seven Brothers*, as I did, and that upon seeing it in 1954, he had made himself some tap shoes and learned all the dances. That at age 17, he'd joined the circus when it came to town, returning home with a new skill – knife throwing – which he practised on his little sisters Tess and Tina.

That at age 22 he'd made a three-tiered revolving wedding cake for his brother Tommy's wedding – as evidenced by an old coloured Kodak slide that my cousin Diana brought to show everyone. And that one of his favourite songs was *Do Not Forsake Me, Oh My Darling* from the movie *High Noon* – also a favourite song of mine.

Shortly afterwards, when I was reviewing my inbox on Facebook Messenger, I read a message from a stranger, which I'd assumed was spam and was about to delete:

> *Dear Jane, I decided I would write to you after reading your writing in memory of Francesco. Frank was a very dear friend of mine and my family for many years. Unfortunately he cut contact with me about 10 years ago. He often spoke of you with great pride and sadness. He built the house I live in, finished now but not by him. My children and I remember him with love. Condolences to you, Juliana and any of his sisters still living. He used to say when he went he wanted God to give him the job of cloud controller, hopefully he got the job. – Suzanne*
>
> *PS I hope one of you got the mirror that had belonged to his mother.*

Suzanne? I had never heard of this person who seemed to know my father in a way that I never did and was telling me what I'd always wanted to hear.

Curious and excited, I replied, asking for more information.

Suzanne, who was the same age as me, told me how they'd met when she had agisted her horse on his property, which she later bought. She'd also met Aunty Mary and Tess and Tina, and Nana's mirror had hung in her house for several years. My father had been part of her family, attending Christmases and birthdays and helping build things. For years they'd met every week to cook a meal and play Scrabble together, and she told me about their conversations:

> *He talked about his parents, siblings and life. He had a great sense of humour and was intelligent in lots of ways, but not so in others.*

I was both fascinated and jealous at this strange normality – the kind of normal that I had missed out on.

However I wasn't surprised that he had eventually cut her off, as he had cut me off and everyone else in his life. She had written to tell me how he felt about me and to seek closure for herself:

> *I missed him very much, but his rejection hurt. He could be very mean, as you and Juliana both know. He was very fragile and used his tongue to protect himself, even when there was no danger. He hated being Italian and what his father had done to him. This created a very insecure man who put people in two camps, those against him and those for him.*

When I told Juliana, she didn't recall ever hearing about Suzanne, but she laughed at the idea of Dad being cloud controller.

"That explains the floods," she said.

I saved Suzanne's message and read it often over the following year and have reproduced parts of it here with her kind permission.

Her words felt both surprising and validating.

Here was a stranger who had given me a rare glimpse of my father: not as the abused son of Gaetano, not as the adored but flawed brother of Tommy, Mary, Tess and Tina, not as the disappointing fool and cruel husband of my mother, not as the neglectful father that I knew, not as the rebellious hero of my sister, not as the crazy creative uncle and stepfather of my cousins, but as a friend – flawed, but loved and valued.

All my life, I had wanted my father to be proud of me, as I had wanted to feel proud of him. Now, I knew. He was proud – and so was I.

Vale, Dad – Francesco (Frank) Ambrogio Maria Bartolomeo Cafarella – whom I will always recognise in my creative and chaotic self, and in all my own dreams, big and small.

Acknowledgements

My grateful thanks to all those who helped bring this story to life.

To my husband, Rob, who listened with endless patience as I relived and pieced together my past over the two intense years of Victorian lockdown during the pandemic.

To Virginia Lloyd, my developmental editor, for her strong guiding hand, and who encouraged me to be the hero of my own story when my focus was still the dreadful story of my mother's betrayal, and who recognised that the real story was "about the sisters".

To my aunts Tess and Tina for telling me the truth about family history, particularly Tess, who supported me during the painful journey of discovery.

To my friend and fellow writer, and former *Age* colleague Marie McNamara for her warm encouragement and for being my first reader outside the family and to Angela Ryan, another friend and fellow writer, for her support and constructive criticism.

To Bradley Dawson, graphic designer and editor at Smith and Brown Design in Castlemaine, who, with respect and compassion, edited and formatted the final version for the PDF that I published on my website, and the many other versions for the many submissions I made to publishers.

To authors Hazel Edwards and Angela Savage, who took time from their busy schedules to read my manuscript and provide generous feedback and endorsements.

To friends and colleagues who read the final draft and provided support and encouragement.

To my children, for letting me write about them – again.

And finally, to my sister, Juliana for her support and courage in allowing me to tell our story.